The Paradigm Lens

Informed Consent to Shared Decision-Making

Steven Kahn

The Paradigm Lens
Informed Consent to Shared Decision-Making
By STEVEN KAHN

ISBN: [979-8-9882552-0-8]
eISBN: [979-8-9882552-1-5]

Cover design by Karp Graphic Design
Formatting by Polgarus Studio

The duck rabbit image is from *Fliegende Blatter* issue 23 October 1892

The Paradigm Lens LLC, Pennsylvania

To Maureen, forever 23-and-pretty – An apropos paradigm
And
Bridget and Alex, our children

Acknowledgments

I wish to acknowledge those who have supported and led me through my various career activities. Bill DeAngelis and Mikael Marlies Karlsson, who let me hang back at Northeastern and learn so much about philosophy. I owe Richard Hull, Peter Hare, and Ken Barber for guiding me through my dissertation on this subject. Jackie Fawcett deserves much credit for conversations and connecting me with the UPenn School of Nursing Health Care Ethics course. The New York State Library for providing the transcript of the Schloendorff trial. Bridget Kahn for helping with some of the figures in the document. My editor Mohamad Al-Hakim for keeping the project on track and being responsive.

Contents

Introduction

My journey to this book began in the 1980s. My dissertation in philosophy centered on informed consent. I saw it as a preliminary work because at the time there weren't a lot of publications concerning rational decision-making under uncertainty, which I believed to be central. It was the beginning of the ascending discipline of behavioral economics, as well as the discipline of bioethics. I loved the interdisciplinary nature of the project. It's stretched from very abstract philosophical points to practical matters.

My career took a similar path. I became a nurse while finishing my dissertation in philosophy. I loved it. It was here that I ran into the realities of the interaction between patients and the health care system from the other side of that equation. I became a member of the hospital's ethics consultation committee. We met with patients, families, and staff to sort out any ethical issues that occurred. As a nurse I faced patients in their real circumstances. I became acutely aware of how poorly informed consent was working. It was a cumbersome activity. Doctors were unsure of what information to give and were inexperienced in how to explain the medical information. Patient self-determination wasn't all that protected or supported. Who knows if the outcomes were good or not. Apparently, I wasn't the only skeptic. Eventually informed consent fell way and shared decision-making (SDM) took its place. Will it suffer the same fate? Will we have to wait more than 50 years to find out?

The aim of this book is to accelerate the development of shared decision-making in health care. The path to that acceleration is to consider informed consent and shared decision-making to be paradigms rather than only theories or models. The word "paradigm" has multiple meanings. Sometimes it can refer to a theory or a model. It can mean a pattern or the prime example of something. In his seminal book *The Structure of Scientific Revolutions,* Thomas

Kuhn investigated many shifts in science through the centuries and treated them as paradigm shifts. He used the term in many senses and in his 1970 second edition said that he would make it more about the fact that a community shares a paradigm and behaves accordingly.

The most useful way to think about paradigms here is to consider the paradigms as providing the world view of the physician and the patient about their interaction. The paradigm offers the people who are having the experience perspectives, tools, and loose boundaries as to what belongs and what doesn't. It involves the way in which the participants tacitly understand how they should behave. It will include models such as decision-making models. It involves disciplines that belong to the topic such as ethics, behavioral economics and by omission leaves out ones that do not. When viewed with this meaning of a paradigm, we can more clearly see why informed consent failed and have a better focus on what shared decision-making should be entertaining as areas of investigation. This would speed up the development of the shared decision-making paradigm, which in turn would help more people. Let us look at the informed consent paradigm.

The simplistic view of the informed consent paradigm is that information flows into the patient's decision-making process, which generates a selection among alternative courses of action. These selections, when followed, generate outcomes. There are different communities of people who study and research the various aspects of this flow. The people involved in the flow are not thinking about paradigms. When I go to the doctor or other health care professional (HCP), I am subconsciously expecting certain behaviors. The purpose of the visit may be to treat and reduce some sort of suffering I have or to do tests to prevent bad things from happening. In short, I believe the HCP has the same goals. The point is to make the most of my health. Now not all the time will we formally discuss a consent. The HCP may say something like "I will take some blood to make a diagnosis." There is no document presented or necessary discussion for me needed. I realize I can say no to this procedure. I can ask questions about the dangers of drawing blood and so on, but I don't. The same is true for blood pressure, listening to my lungs and other non-invasive activities.

Even here, we can make some caveats as to what is to follow. Much of the time we don't really go through procedures for obtaining consent to do things, as the patient may already be experienced in the normal practice of a physician visit. There are times, though, that the process is understood to be necessary. Where informing becomes essential to protect self-determination. There always are paradigms at play, so to speak. The first is the paradigm of the health care situation and seeking out an HCP to help. I am, for purposes of brevity, going to refer to the purpose of the health care visit as to make the patient as well as possible. Medical decisions should be made with this goal in mind. The other goal, or restriction for some, is to respect patient self-determination. Whatever the paradigm, it must look to both goals, and as ethics may dictate sacrifice the medical condition in order to respect self-determination.

In the end informed consent as a paradigm failed because it treated information improperly. Consequently, it neither protected patients' self-determination nor promoted good medical outcomes (President's Commission, Katz). The paradigm shifted to shared decision-making and a focus on the patient participating more in the decision process. Exactly how they are to participate is vague. Somehow it would seem after negotiating with each other, the patient and HCP both agree. I know that is not true all the time. It might not even be true more than 75 percent of the time. Furthermore, there is plenty of research into information and delivery, especially since the Affordable Care Act was passed making SDM a more likely approach. Glyn Elwyn has worked on this extensively and a good summary appears in Elwyn (2021).

As you read through this book, it helps to consider the various parts of the paradigm. Information exchange is part of both paradigms. It remains a pivotal point in the maturation process of SDM. Ethics certainly has a role. After all, the requirement of respecting self-determination (sometimes referred to as autonomy in this context) is based on which ethical theory you adopt. The boundaries of this respect can shift because of the choice of ethical theory. Decision-making models play a significant role in two ways. The model of choice needs to process the information provided and produce reasonably good outputs. Also, our ability as humans to implement the decision-making (DM) model needs to be proficient enough to get to reasonably good solutions.

Each of these will have its own specifics to flesh out. Here are a few items:

- The DM model will need to account for facts and values—very different data types.
- Decision makers need to be able to prioritize their values.
- Decision makers need to be able to place a value on an outcome and compare values.

Chapter 1 begins with discussing paradigms in more detail. If you like analogies, then think of a paradigm as a way of looking at a world. Here the world is of an HCP patient visit or encounter. When we are in it, we are stakeholders interacting with the lens of the paradigm upon our very noses. We are not surprised with how others act in the situations so long as we are all versed in the paradigm behavior.

Chapter 2 introduces dining out as a paradigm which is instructive as to how information is pivotal to self-determination or power. Now we generally don't use these words when we are dining out. They don't form part of that paradigm. Yet using a distant activity provides a useful perspective. The role of information in controlling one's decisions becomes all so evident. There is a migration of legal cases where a new challenge of informing piles on in each subsequent case. Similarly, we develop the dining examples. The root cause of the failure is reason enough to shift paradigms. The problems with informing in the court decisions are well documented (King 437-446). Patient information is necessary, and not just any patient information.

In Chapter 3 we review the prevalent DM models. Each DM model places constraints on the information required by the model to process the information appropriately. A good process will provide better outcomes for the patient. It will also be a necessary condition for having the right to self-determination. Patients need some level of competency when they use the process to have the right to self-determination.

Whatever decision-making model is chosen, including my current favorite, it will face obstacles of our human limitations. The adaption of the Goldilocks fable gives us some ideas about experience and its relation to establishing preferences. Behavioral Economics as a discipline has uncovered numerous biases and mistakes in our ways of processing information. We survey what is most relevant for these types of decisions. The SDM paradigm will need to address with empirical studies what works best for people to enhance their decision-making prowess.

The ethics underlying the self-determination requirement is then brought to the fore in Chapter 4 through two famous cases in Bioethics. The chapter provides support for the idea of the practical importance and is meant to tug at your intuitions. Part of the reason for the detail here is that my own practical experience is that situations for consent are far from the pristine abstractions provided in most texts. Discussions in seminars with students reinforced the idea that a lot can be learned about what is relevant when looking at all the circumstances. Most cases will tug on you in more than one direction.

Earlier we mentioned that ethics plays a role in all of this. It underlies the whole paradigm, really. This is not the place to provide a course on the two main ethical theory types, but in Chapter 5 we give a very truncated version of consequentialist and deontological approaches. There we present some of the ways that ethical theory and thinking plays into the arguments we see in in the adoption of the paradigm.

Chapter 5 includes other philosophical considerations to be explored. We noted the vital role of competency. Over the years I have witnessed and participated in too many conflations of the concept of competency. How we interpret competency will determine the way we defend or oppose the idea of someone's competency. How competent do you have to be to be self-determining? Likewise, as HCPs how do we help someone reach that level?

An interesting feature of the discussions in Chapter 5 is that the most people have focused the decision-making under uncertainty with respect to a person's current preference. We know that we change over time including how we order our preferences. But what about my future self who must live with the results? Interesting philosophical notions.

Chapter 6 is the concluding chapter which looks at how we might progress from here. There exist numerous pieces of research that involve health literacy and the like, all of which needs to be more explicitly integrated into the paradigm. I leave it off there as my current state of investigation which I hope prompts others to further clarify, discover and properly discard notions I have set forward to move this bar more quickly.

The Appendices are reserved for those who like more technical details. Appendix A is meant for Philosophy majors or those with equivalent masochistic tendencies. It is an argument for the proper place of "can" in competency. It is a way of involving the concept of "success" in determining competency. Appendix B is a more thorough discussion of cardinal rankings and shows us one way we actually combine differing values. It demonstrates a bit of the arbitrary nature of the enterprise. Appendix C is a mathematical formulation of Expected Value or Utility. These are meant as guides for the type of depth I think is required to fill in the paradigm in a meaningful way. They may simply be of interest to you, as they were to me.

Chapter 1

The Paradigm Lens

Imagine you just walked into a dining establishment. You are seated, and a menu is presented to you. The staff departs, and you begin looking through the menu. Meanwhile, a server comes out and places a bowl of chili directly in front of you. Your response might be, "I haven't placed any order yet. This must be for someone else." At this point, the waitstaff responds, "This is what you are getting. We don't take orders here."

Well, at the very least, this feels odd. We all have an idea in mind of what to expect when we enter a restaurant, and this is not it. This is not the expected causal order of things. We generally expect to place a food order first and then be served. This always involves food or beverages. Somewhere in the process, a bill comes, and we pay. We can think of this as a paradigm.

Our reaction to the above scenario is due to the actions of the server not meeting expectations. What counts as acceptable behavior at a restaurant is culturally determined to some extent. The world of restaurant dining is interpreted through a paradigm lens. It is not the same paradigm as other dining experiences. For example, when friends invite you over for dinner, normally, you will not get a bill and be expected to pay (okay, my friends might give me one, but that is another issue altogether).

The world of restaurant dining is one domain. Its little world is populated by food, beverage, people, money, and so on. The view we have of that world is a paradigm. The word "paradigm" itself has multiple meanings. Our focus will be on the notion of a paradigm as a worldview.

A fascinating feature of these worldviews is that you can have more than one paradigm lens for the same world. The cover of this book contains a famous ambiguous figure—the duck/rabbit. There is no question that the illustration is one drawing, but we can perceive it in two distinct ways. We can look at it as a duck paradigm, so to speak, with a bill to the left. We can also see it as a rabbit with its ears to the left. Reality is influenced by the paradigm through which we visualize it. The paradigm can be thought of as a lens. It will block out extraneous data. In the case of the duck-rabbit illustration, when looking for the rabbit, we're going to look for the ears. It's the hallmark feature of a rabbit. Indeed, if I had instructed you to look for the ears of the figure, it would be unlikely for you to see the duck's bill. Paradigm lenses bring certain items into focus while filtering others out.

The first time I became acquainted with the concept of a paradigm was while reading Thomas Kuhn's *The Structure of Scientific Revolutions*. It had a rather profound effect on my thinking. It was one of those works that captivate you while you argue against it. I had a rather firm belief in the forward march of science toward knowledge and truth. Experiments were required to support hypotheses, which in the end, would both predict and explain how everything worked. At some intuitive level, I still believe in this general idea.

However, it has become clear to me that this march is anything but steady or necessarily forward moving when you describe what occurs in science. One of the primary assumptions for believing in this progress is that the data from experiments are independent of the theories and paradigms supporting them—or the individual interpreting them. Kuhn's darn book made it exceedingly difficult to show that the observations are independent of theories and that they are absolutely neutral in proving the theories to be either true or false. This reality has tamped my enthusiasm for a completely independent set of facts to support a theory. The relationship between what we see and think to our paradigms is like wearing rose-colored lenses. The lens makes everything appear as a red hue. Does the real world contain nothing but red objects? If we are wedded to a paradigm, we can only see those things that the paradigm allows us to see.

We utilize paradigms to train individuals in various activities.

Teaching is a good example. We include materials for class presentation in the training, homework, syllabus, and several other aids. Unless it is a training session in metal fabrication, we are unlikely to include welding in the curriculum.

Paradigms can be judged as to whether they accomplish their purpose. Typically, a paradigm will shift when it has trouble completing the task and goals it has set for itself. Usually, this happens when confronting a particularly sticky problem. The sociology and history of those changes are interesting. As to why the new paradigm is accepted over the old one, the answer is hazy. The rationale for making the shift was not based on improved predictive or explanatory power. A more recent paradigm handled the problem that the older one could not. Sometimes it was more elegant in its approach.

The history of the phlogiston theory is a splendid example (Conant 69-74). Phlogiston was originally conceived as a substance that existed either in the heat of a flame or in matter. Observers noted that when you place wood in a fire, it becomes ash. What happened to all that other stuff that made up the wood? The phlogiston was driven out. An anomaly to this idea happened when you heated certain metals. Instead of losing weight, they gained weight. How the chemists at that time tried to handle this sticky problem was to claim that phlogiston had a negative weight (Conant 72). What people will not do to save their favorite paradigm.

Many problems occur when one practices within a paradigm. It loses its force as a paradigm when these sticky problems remain glued to it. In science, these would typically be called anomalies. They may only upend a theory or a paradigm when the anomaly does not go away elegantly. Rather than giving us a unified view of the world, the anomalies receive patches.

A Health Care Paradigm: Autonomy and Good Decision-Making

We will be approaching informed consent and shared decision-making from the standpoint of the two paradigms. One is grounded in respecting patient autonomy, and the other is in making good decisions. If a paradigm does not accomplish autonomy and good decision-making goals, we will have a sticky problem. As is the case with other paradigm shifts, there is a puzzle that cannot

9

be solved from within the paradigm. However, the shift to shared decision-making (SDM) is meant to solve that puzzle. We will inspect the lens of each paradigm for its imperfections. Notably, there is an intuitive grasp of what was wrong with informed consent. Moreover, shared decision-making enabled a solution to that problem. This is typical of paradigm shifts. People grasp the problem and shift the focus without a root cause analysis of what went wrong in the first place.

Informed consent failed to protect patient rights (President's Commission 29-36). Several issues were noted in legal cases as portrayed below. As with any paradigm, it takes some time for the practitioners to seek a solution. Court cases extend in the US back to the 1800s, and the cases really accelerated in the mid-20th century. The information needed was a critical element in protecting patient rights. The ethical literature also saw an upsurge since 1970 around the issues of consent and the principle of respecting individual autonomy. Journals and centers such as the *Hastings Center Report*, *The Journal of Medical Ethics* and the Kennedy Center's Bioethics Research Library had their beginnings in the decade.

To get started, we need to be more explicit about the concept of a paradigm as it can have various meanings. For example, it can be a philosophical framework from which generalizations and experiments are performed. Or it can be an outstandingly clear or typical example of something. It can also mean a way of looking at things.

We will adopt the last meaning for our purpose. It includes the notion of a worldview or framework. As with the duck-rabbit illustration, there is a pattern there. You would recognize a broad range of completions of the rest of the body as a duck or rabbit. The duck would have webbed feet. Or you could imagine the image being a mother duck with the baby ducks following behind. We can identify numerous variations of duck.

On the other hand, you would be shocked if the rabbit had webbed feet. The rabbit pattern does not include webbed feet. The way in which we imagine rabbits excludes webbed feet. It also excludes some behavior patterns that ducks exhibit—e.g., baby ducks following a line behind a mother duck. Rabbits do not behave that way.

Observing a world through a paradigm's lens will generate certain expectations. It will establish the types of things to expect and other things that will be a shock if seen. The world that is under observation, in large measure dictates the types of things that belong and the types that do not.

Paradigms can have a variety of elements. The illustration consists of visual elements that are under consideration. The paradigms will also apply when looking at live objects. They will also have the sounds and behaviors that ducks and rabbits exhibit. These paradigms are successful because we can distinguish between ducks and rabbits. That is the goal of the paradigm.

Paradigms can be successes or failures. The criteria used for judging success and failure depend upon the type of world being observed. Our paradigms for rabbits and ducks work quite well out in the wild. We can distinguish one from the other. But informed consent is a trickier enterprise. It is not only sights and sounds that we are naming, but behaviors as well. These behaviors are constructs to attain goals. First, the behaviors include protecting patient autonomy. The behaviors are meant to promote patient self-determination. We need to employ more than our five senses to do this.

There is a derivative goal as well, namely, we want to make good decisions. Now, this latter goal may be related to a different paradigm. The medical encounter itself is trying to either prevent, mitigate, or cure a problem. Both goals are meant to succeed. Many ethical debates in medicine revolve around issues of meeting both goals simultaneously. Paternalistic interventions were predominant when the second goal superseded the first. The law allowed the HCP to be paternalistic when the patient does not possess sufficient decision-making capacity.

The rationale is that the patient cannot make good decisions or will not make good decisions. This carve-out, which seems intuitive, needs to be accounted for in the models. Ethical components make their way into informed consent and shared decision-making as part of the paradigm. Typically, it is not made explicit. It is assumed as the raison d'être for the activity to exist. Both goals will be required to be met by the paradigm.

If you observed an informed consent encounter in 1980, you would be able to describe the pattern that allows you to identify it as an informed consent activity. You would see the physician talking to the patient about their diagnosis and what the doctor recommends as a course of action. If it involved surgery, a document was printed outlining the various and sundry pitfalls that might happen. They were written in medical jargon for the most part. Patients were not expected to ask questions. Once the patient orally approved and/or signed the form, the activity was over. I experienced this as a patient, nurse, and ethics consultant.

Informed consent in medical research has its twists and turns. The paradigms involved in that area were codified by the WMA with the Declaration of Helsinki in 1964. The latest version has some significant changes (Declaration). The very notion of the informed consent paradigm was involved and focused on removing coercion and generating full disclosure. Subsequent versions spelled out several things to be disclosed. The reading level of the informed consent document came into focus. Formal proof of obtaining subject/patient signatures gained importance.

With a shift in paradigms to shared decision-making in health care, there was also a change in what was studied by researchers in connection with the shift. Research continued in the area of writing comprehensible text for patients. Shared decision-making would demand more. Pharmaceutical studies would be transferred from a physician-mediated paradigm to a patient-centered one. My experience working in pharmaceutical research from 1991on was the incorporation of data directly from patients into reports. The most recent example of this would be the FDA allowing direct patient reporting to be considered valuable evidence in evaluating a drug's efficacy and safety profile. Indeed, it is remarkable to note how much the words "patient-centered" are now used. Resources have now shifted toward ways of obtaining patient information directly without the use of investigator sites. This has also led to an increase in technology in regulatory parameters in these studies. From my history of being involved with setting up research studies, it has gone from a pure paper investigator type of research through an intermediate period where information was collected from both the physicians and the patients directly. I can tell you that combining that data was more than a little bit of a challenge. This last leg of the shift has been to decrease information from physicians and allow patients to send along their medical records for abstraction and patient-reported outcomes. These reported outcomes may involve questionnaires that have been rigorously tested for validity.

On the health care side, the shift has been more about the research into supporting patient value discovery and the manner of transmitting the information. The research has moved toward the environment of the information exchange and the media used. Is it better in person or via video? How about written documentation and links to websites? Academic institutions formed to study these issues, including the Center for Shared Decision-making DHMC and Clinics. Even though the term "shared decision-making"has been around since 1982, it received a boost with the passage of the Affordable Care Act in the United States (Patient Protection and Affordable Care Act 2010). The hope was that patients were more likely to participate in their therapy if there was a discussion and the decision-making was shared. Besides this laudable goal was the additional one of improving decision quality and reducing costs. Money was set aside through the Act to study ways to promote shared decision-making in medical practice.

From my experience as a nurse and serving on an ethics consultation committee in a major hospital, most of the issues faced by patients and staff were around communication and not ethical quagmires. Most of the time, it involved at least one of the parties not listening to the other. People were talking past each other. The importance of communication may even lead to a significantly different approach to informed consent (Manson).

We will rest on a focal point as we develop our paradigm lens.

Paradigms are very instructive. When you work within a paradigm, whether it be chemistry or medical practice, or nursing practice, certain expectations are created within it. The universe of activities and experiences you anticipate is governed through that lens. We expect controlled experiments, equations, references to atoms, and so on in chemistry. A new paradigm in the field may lend itself to abandoning the notion of the elements. A great example of a scientific revolution involved abandoning the phlogiston theory in favor of the oxygen theory of gases. After that paradigm transition, phlogiston became extinct. It ceased to be part of the vocabulary of chemistry. Chemists soon stopped talking about phlogiston or experimenting with it, except for a few stragglers, such as Joseph Priestley. Old proponents tend to die off. From a sociological point of view or even a historical perspective, no one tries to prove that phlogiston does not exist anymore. The group that works in chemistry has adopted a new paradigm. The new paradigm offered new insights into how gases would work, involving careful weighing and quantitating the results of experiments. The new theory predicted these results, whereas the old theory would not predict how much more or less something would weigh after burning. This information was not even on the radar.

When put this way, various problems of social interactions lend themselves to new insights when you adopt a new paradigm. In this case, we are specifically looking at the paradigms of informed consent and shared decision-making in medical practice. These paradigms have certain goals as part of their paradigm. Similar to the sciences, whose goals are prediction and explanation, our paradigms have the goals of respecting autonomy and making good decisions. The success and failure of informed consent as a paradigm can be judged according to how well or poorly it meets these goals. It does poorly and we have a series of court cases to prove the point. Each new case tries to plug a gap discovered in the paradigm.

It starts with the information being provided to the patient. As new cases arose, the courts were compelled to figure out new ways to apply the paradigm. This is because the patients' rights were not being respected in each case. Yet the prior rulings did not address this issue when new circumstances arose. Each subsequent ruling plugged in the holes. This left the whole edifice somewhat structurally unsound. The question is, why did this happen?

Uncovering the reasons for these failures from a conceptual point of view reveals a need for more understanding of how decision-making works. Each case does build a little bit and provides more protection for the patient. It never gets to what I consider the root cause of the issue: the lack of patient participation in the information exchange. When we unpack the details of decision-making in this context, we find that the existing decision-making models would warrant more patient participation. It also speaks to what types of information the patient needs to provide in the process.

Historically, a certain model of rational decision-making has been somewhat assumed by writers on the topic (Tversky s251). It was considered the normative or ideal. This model has also entered into the ethics of the decision-making process (Thornton 1099). The connection between the decision, the decision-making capacity, and ethics can be found as early as the 1912 case of Schloendorff v. the Society of New York hospital. In that case in the appeals court, Judge Cardozo stated that all adults of a sound mind have the right to do what they want with their bodies. The sound mind connects the right to decision-making capacity. In fact, much of the paternalistic discussions around not allowing patients to make their own decisions often invoke the idea that patients do not have the decision-making capacity to make proper choices.

Historically, the gold standard of a decision-making model under uncertainty has been the expected value or the expected utility model. Either of those models assumes the nature of the information that needs to be supplied for processing. As I will show, the information required for making a good choice differs from the information these two models require. We need something different.

Some reject the notion that expected utility is the best rational approach in a number of scenarios. Gerd Gigerenzer is one of the most prominent of those who offers an alternative model of decision-making (Gigerenzer 2008). We shall explore Gigerenzer's approach along with another alternative steeped in philosophy's past —Bentham's approach to utilitarianism, albeit somewhat adapted to our purposes. These offer better solutions since they allow for other types of information to be integrated into the decision-making apparatus. The Expected Value/Utility model fails for sure, and that leaves these two still in play.

There are numerous challenges still left to overcome. People still must be able to process probabilities in some measure and be less subjected to pernicious biases. This is no easy task. As it turns out, these challenges hold true regardless of who's making the decision. Physicians, statisticians, and the lay public are all subject to these biases in our thinking. For a number of these, there are ways to guard ourselves against going down the wrong road and making good decisions. The latter chapters try to organize these challenges and yield methods for dealing with them.

So let us proceed with some of the methodologies in use here—examples, which in and of themselves do not bring pernicious bias with them. For the legal cases, we are going to take the paradigm of dining where life and death struggles, hopefully, are not at the fore. The use of examples has a history in academic philosophy.

Throughout the book there are some fictitious cases engineered to grab at our intuitions. A rather famous example of using a fictitious case is that of Judith Thomson, who created a scenario she leveraged for arguments about abortion (Thomson 27-46). Briefly, Thomson offers a scenario involving two individuals having their circulatory systems linked together so that one can survive. As she put it, imagine that you wake up one morning to find that you're hooked up to a concert violinist; if you separate from them, they will die. You did not ask for it, but you're saddled with it. This is analogous to the issue of being pregnant because of rape. Most people believe you do not have to stay hooked to that violinist. Even the segment of the population that believes abortion is wrong under all circumstances believes that you should be able to remove yourself from the violinist. This is what I discovered in the classroom. Such cases make us see that we do have conflicting intuitions that beg for a justification. Alas, they don't prove much beyond our own conceptual conflicts. They do, however, highlight that we need to make hard choices in order to be consistent. More importantly, they bring to the front the essence of what needs to be explored. In short, these cases improve our understanding of the issues.

The approach taken in this book aims to first ensure that we understand what is going on. I like to draw on examples from other areas of life to help illustrate the arguments, such as the opening diner paradigm example. These examples tell us much about communication. They are not meant to prove points. We are starting with the assumption that people have the right to make their own decisions. We will not be proving that point. From time to time, philosophy texts will resort to fictional concoctions to prove a point relying on the reader having similar intuitions.

It is critical to note that the only certain result from this example is that you have two intuitions that really do not say what you need to do or how to resolve the conflict, or which one is the right one. For those individuals who believe abortion is wrong in every case, however, they must agree that the violinist has no right to her body. You are obligated to support them, or they have to come up with another reason why you could detach yourself from the violinist, but the mother is not allowed to detach herself from the fetus. Similarly, the diner examples below appeal to our intuitions in a more straightforward context where our emotions and biases sometimes will cloud the example. The consequences clearly are entirely different. The idea is that the same principles would apply to the communication required.

The challenge is a question of what we are to do with these opposing intuitions. It is so easy to overstep how far one should go. The fact that some people have contradictory intuitions does not mean or indicate which of the two is correct. It only shows that people who are opposed to abortion in all circumstances need to be able to come up with some reasoning that shows what is distinct between the two cases. Reason will always have to come along at some point. Our intuitions are not necessarily infallible.

Nevertheless, the examples illustrate that there may be a problem with how one interprets situations based on personal intuitions. Typically, the philosophical approach attempts to pull out what is important and leave behind what is not. This is my approach to the use of these examples. We will be relying initially on the diner, which is not fraught with ethical complications, to examine the information-sharing activity. In some sense, it will serve us well.

Chapter 2

Recipe for Failure

The Paradigm Diner

Welcome to the Paradigm Diner. I know you were expecting something about informed consent or shared decision-making, or patient rights. It will come soon enough.

For now, imagine your prototypical diner from the outside. The chrome façade reflects the sunlight beautifully. The neon lights project that familiar glow of color combinations not usually chosen to coexist. If you have experienced dining in such a facility, you will already be harboring certain expectations of what should greet you when you enter.

You have brought a few friends and hope to get a booth. As the three of you step inside, the "Wait to be Seated" sign immediately hits you, clearly serving its purpose well. A staff member approaches and inquires, "For four? Booth or table?"

"Booth."

The hostess leads you around the corner and you are seated. Paper napkins support the silverware. A wait staff member shows up and says she needs some help to serve us. Whereupon she calls for a colleague who comes with a plate of mashed potatoes. The first server holds your head while the second takes a handful of the potatoes and slops it on your face.

Presumably, you, too, find this behavior reprehensible. Shocking really. It fails to meet the standards of proper etiquette. It certainly takes you aback because it is not what you expect to happen in a diner. Typically, after being seated, you get your menu, place an order, get served, dine, and pay at the register. That is the paradigm of eating at a diner.

Well, you might think this is an interesting example, but are probably wondering what it has to do, if anything, with informed consent? Indeed, no doctor or other health care professional (HCP) behaves this way. Hopefully, not anymore. But let us go back to the documented beginning of informed consent in the law. Unfortunately, such a case exists.

Slater v Baker and Stapleton: A Case of Callous Treatment

Let us visit the first informed consent case. This is an unfortunate case whereby Mr. Slater sued Dr. Baker and Stapleton for receiving poor medical care rather than for lack of gaining his consent (Slater v Baker and Stapleton 860- 863). The case is depicted here from the court record.

Mr. Slater, in 1766 or thereabouts, had suffered a fall and broke his leg. He was attended to by a surgeon. The surgeon testified that after a month, a callous had formed with a small protuberance which was not unusual. The patient stayed with Latham, an apothecary, through much of his recovery. After nine weeks, Latham sent him on his way back home. According to Latham, Mr. Slater was well enough to go home. His bones had sufficiently mended (united).

That Slater was doing well at this point was corroborated by another witness who stated that when he came home from his stay with Latham, Slater could walk with crutches. So, we have the testimony of his status that he was doing well and healing when he came home.

At this point, neither Baker nor Stapleton have entered the scene. Why were they involved? The court records show that Mr. Slater invited Stapleton, another apothecary, to come for the express purpose of removing the bandages. As best as I can determine, Stapleton, after he arrived and looked at the leg, told Mr. Slater that he wanted some help and requested Dr. Baker, a surgeon, to join him in the endeavor.

It is important to take a moment here and imagine us in this situation from Slater's vantage point. You're at home after nine weeks. Why was Stapleton sending for a doctor when everything was going well? You must be wondering if something is wrong. Stapleton had asked you if it would be OK to have Doctor Baker assist. Really? How hard is it to take off a bandage and replace it? You acquiesce. How many of us would feel similarly? It is hard to put yourself in the place of somebody in 18th-century London but being confronted with a medical situation is not so foreign to us.

Baker arrived with a machine with steel teeth in it. Now, if I had seen this contraption, I think I would start asking some questions. "Is that some sort of experimental piece of hardware?" "What are you going to do with that thing?" There is no indication in the court testimony that Slater objected to any of this. The ensuing description of events indicates that there were prior discussions between Stapleton and Baker before they arrived on the scene. Stapleton took Slater's broken leg and placed it upon his knee. He applied the metal contraption with its teeth. He got a nod from Baker, and Stapleton proceeded to crack the knee and break the callous that had formed. Immediately upon the force of Stapleton's action, Slater let out an exclamation, and I quote, "You have broken what nature formed!" I would have slightly different phrasing for my scream, and it is something that should not appear in this book.

This certainly feels wrong. It is eerily like the diner example. In both cases, I need to be made aware of what will happen, although there are some clues. The clues, notwithstanding, are not a substitute for informing me exactly what's going to happen. Either case is wrong. This establishes the connection between information and ethics. Are there other intuitions we might have about this case?

Amazingly enough, there is an alternative source for the facts contrasting with those that appear in the court record (Miller 1-4). It also fills in many gaps in the court record and makes corrections to it. Will this alter our intuition about the case?

A summary of Baker's notes to his hospital serves up a somewhat different picture.

Slatter (correct spelling) fell from a horse and broke his tibia and fibula with an upper and lower break in each bone. He was attended to by the Lathams, a father and son who were both surgeons and apothecaries. Slatter stayed with one of them for those nine weeks.

Once home, Slatter called Stapleton (now also a surgeon) because he was having "discomfort with the bandage." A somewhat different flavor than needing a bandage change. As before, Stapleton arrived and determined that the situation was more difficult for him to manage alone. The upper fracture was located toward the knee, but the lower one looked uncertain to him. There was a small protuberance from it.

Slatter wanted Baker in the case not only because he wanted a second opinion, but he had determined that it was not as well healed as he was led to believe. Here is where the number of visits is given in a bit more detail. During their initial visit, Baker and Stapleton redressed the leg. Neither felt it was healing well. This was reinforced by the fact that Slatter was having pain. This pain did not come out in the court record. Baker had decided to put a brace on the leg before they came back. Oh, so that is the terrible steel thing with teeth. It is not an experimental device to lengthen or shorten the leg. It was a new type of brace. And to beat all, Slatter did not yell out at that time about the brace. He was not crazy about it either, as he stopped using it before the doctors returned.

The night before the next appointment, Slatter's daughter contacted Stapleton and informed him that Slatter was in a great deal of pain. Apparently, he tried to put weight on the leg and messed it up even more. Stapleton just bandaged it again and returned with Baker the next day.

When they arrived, Slatter wanted to know what they could do about reducing the protuberance, and both Baker and Stapleton agreed that they would have to break the callous and reset the leg. Here is the key point. Slatter refused. Baker and Stapleton came back for the third time, and after Baker gently tried to reset the leg, he went ahead and broke his leg (reduced the fracture) when Slatter's voice gave rise to the quote above.

I have different feelings about the participants depending on the version of the case. After reading the first (court) version, I found myself filling in the gaps. The brace felt experimental and was not described as a brace. I mistakenly felt it played a role in the pain he suffered. Also, not reading about the fact that Slatter (Slater) walked on the leg to make it worse seemed to soften my reaction but did not change it. After all, Baker and Stapleton still did something they were told not to do, which might even be worse than acting without informing at all.

In either case, their actions were wrong. The court-recorded version resembles the diner example. It shows us that valid consent requires some information. At the very least, it requires information about what is going to be done.

Even though our intuitions are strong on these descriptions of the Slater case, some arguments might sway our intuitions. In reviewing the case, it is possible to hypothesize that Slater gave tacit consent for the procedure. According to the court version, he did see the device and did not comment on it. Probably, he could figure out that they were going to attach it to his leg. By not objecting, he was giving tacit consent to the procedure.

A tacit consent, or any expressed consent, would require more information about what is about to happen. The contraption may have been viewed as a brace by Slater and not a breaking of the leg. At most, one could reasonably surmise that he did not object to putting the contraption on the leg. Nothing is stated in the court-recorded version about signals for rebreaking the leg. As Baker's notes revealed, Slater actually told them (Baker and Stapleton) not to break his leg the day before.

It is a straightforward case from a consent point of view. Most of the subsequent examples are far more complicated. The information requirements go beyond the basic "this is what we will be doing." As the subsequent examples demonstrate, the right information gives us more control over attaining our goals. We are not shooting in the dark.

What is the informed consent paradigm? What lenses are we required to put on? Is that the right prescription? The answer depends upon the context. This can be attributed to the several meanings and references of the concept. It can refer to the practice of obtaining valid informed consent through a discussion. It also refers to a signed document detailing benefits and risks, usually surgical. It was developed over a few centuries as a practice to protect patient rights and/or secure patient compliance. As a legal construct, the informed consent paradigm is meant to secure the patient's right to self-determination. In the court system, several seminal cases continued to articulate the paradigm as previous versions were found wanting. Each subsequent case displayed an attempt to plug the holes left by prior decisions. Eventually, the paradigm was found to be lacking. At a certain point, you want to build a new paradigm, as the repairs to the old one leaves you feeling there is not enough structural integrity left worth saving.

A new paradigm was initiated in an attempt to resolve the issues presented in informed consent. That paradigm is Shared Decision-making (SDM). So let us see why the informed consent paradigm failed. Perhaps it can instruct us on how to build the SDM paradigm.

The interaction between the health care provider and the patient is also a social activity. The informed consent model provided patients with protection for making health care decisions. It was one of those phrases that "sounds good in theory" but is rather difficult to put into practice. Like other practices, these gave us guideposts for the activities we should expect from the participants. The success or failure of the paradigm for this social activity in health care is if it protects patient autonomy and promotes good health care decisions. This means we will judge the informed consent paradigm and any other paradigm competing with it based on how well it would protect patient autonomy and support good decision-making. The method I have chosen for judging informed consent is to leverage court cases that have already occurred. Historically these cases have a natural progression in them. They keep finding additional problems and holes with prior decisions. Each build on the prior, but they never seem to get to the essence of the failure. It turns out that each patch results in a less-than-systematic paradigm. The reason for the failure may seem simple once we go through the cases. It just goes to show you that if you're looking for something, it is easier to find it. The book's first section is devoted to uncovering the essential flaw in the informed consent paradigm.

This brings us to the question of what the informed consent paradigm is. Let us start with a rough outline of the expected activities. The starting point for the paradigm is when the patient has described their symptoms and the HCP has evaluated any signs and typically diagnostic tests, though even the tests may require consent if they are not typical. So let us mark this as the starting point when the HCP gives the patient some information. They performed some assessments, which offered up a diagnosis. The diagnosis itself has a likely set of outcomes if not treated. Like you are "likely to feel worse over the next few months. The disease may leave you with a residual effect of having difficulty breathing," and so on. To mitigate against these outcomes, certain interventions may be offered that require consent. The HCP will then provide the information about the intervention. It is hard to say what is typical in the information package. Details surrounding the likelihood of success, or the level of success may be in there or not. Risks associated with the intervention are typically to be expected. The patient then signs off, literally or figuratively, on the choice. That is the paradigm for informed consent, be it very roughly.

The paradigm was meant to accomplish two goals, as you may recall. It was there to protect the patient's right to decide. This was paramount in the law because the cases revolved around this point of rights. The other goal is to supply information so that the patient can make the best possible decision for themselves. Evaluating the paradigm's success or failure should be based on how well it accomplishes meeting these two goals.

What is particularly noteworthy is that people had clear ideas as to what criteria were not met by the old paradigm. The dissemination of information was highly variable, with hospitalized patients receiving little information (President's Commission 80). Clinical study consent forms were at a college reading level (Baker 2646-2648). Patient compliance with the medical decisions was not good (Greenberg 592-599). The question of why the informed consent model was not working had not become an issue until the late 1970s. Informed consent documents were not at a reading level that an eighth grader could understand. Okay, but that does not mean the paradigm is faulty as much as the implementation needs to be more careful. Nevertheless, the shift away from the informed consent paradigm started in the late 1970s, and it was eventually replaced with the shared decision-making paradigm in the Affordable Care Act (ACA) here in the US (this is not the case in the law, where informed consent remains the legal doctrine).

The goal here is to protect patient rights and promote better patient outcomes. Naturally, we will look at how informed consent failed to bring about either or both outcomes. In 1982 the President's Commission published its Making Health Care Decisions, which noted that informed consent missed several practical items. Patients did not seem to receive a significant amount of the information., especially surrounding risks (President's Commission). There was also evidence that the lack of compliance could be related to how much patients participated in the conversation or if they had been given information. Other studies have further reinforced this. One differential component of the SDM model is that the patient engages in the decision-making and, consequently, is theoretically more likely to comply with treatment. Compliance is important in attaining the best health outcomes. The prime motivation for the shift at the time was ethical. People realized that the discussions surrounding standards of informing were not leading to protection of patient self-determination.

The pivot from the informed consent paradigm to the shared decision-making paradigm is an interesting shift. There needs to be a comprehensive analysis of why the informed consent paradigm failed. It is prudent to look at the factors that led to its downfall comprehensively before running off to a new paradigm. You will likely repeat some of the same mistakes if you are not aware of what went wrong. As for SDM, it is not easy even to figure out what the paradigm is, to be honest. There is no standard definition of shared decision-making other than information shared. Sometimes the actual choice looks like it might be a unanimous vote by the stakeholders. This is a laudable goal, but it feels a little bit Pollyanna-ish. Given that there will occasionally be disagreements between the physician and patient, there must be a final arbiter of the therapy selection.

The problem with the vagueness surrounding the paradigm for shared decision-making is that it does not guide the health care provider or the patient. What information is relevant for sharing will remain unclear. How to package the information and explain its importance is still problematic. Exactly what is the patient bringing to the table?

Some issues are typically brought up in discussions and papers about SDM. Often, they involve patient comprehension of the medical information. It is obvious that the information needs to be something we comprehend to be at all useful. Is that enough? No, as you will read in the upcoming chapters, it is not. Other elements are missing, and I believe we have been missing them because we have not pulled together the underlying goals of informed consent. The ethics of the situation drives some of it, and the realities of how we think as humans play an essential role. The history of informed consent and medical ethics bears this out. Informed consent loses its prominence as a social practice (except for legal practice) because it does not get us to the goals of protecting autonomy or improving outcomes. Shared decision-making feels like it should help achieve both goals, though it does not address all the issues explicitly. The hidden variable in all of this is the decision-making model. It forms the basis of what skill sets we need as decision-makers and the types of information we require to make good decisions.

As a spoiler alert, the fault lies with the presumed model of rationality, which is either the Expected Value or Expected Utility model. It is hard to live up to the constraints of either model. These models of rationality play a role in determining patient competency (decision-making capacity), which is the condition for autonomy and the patient's right to make the choice. They also dictate what types of information are needed to make a good decision. These models will fail because they require information which does not align with the information used in this type of decision. They also fail on one other count. They are too hard for humans to perform well. We are notoriously poor at making the required calculations. Both aspects are explored below.

Consent Is Needed

This linkage between consent and information is enshrined originally in Slater. The consent itself is a requirement and confers an obligation on the part of the physician to let the patient make the decision. Slater illustrates that information is a necessary component to protect autonomy. Though we will be concentrating on this informational aspect, for the time being, it is important to note that the ability to make decisions is another essential element.

The first instance of connecting autonomy and the ability to decide can be found in Schloendorff v The Society of The NY Hospital. Judge Cardozo proclaim that every adult of sound mind has the right to make their own decision. He forged the link between the soundness of mind and age with an ethical right. We should characterize it as a legal right as well. We will be investigating this case in detail later. From both Slater and Schloendorff, we can conclude that the patient's right to make a choice is connected both to the information needed and their ability to make decisions.

The right to make the decision inevitably leads to a short discussion about rights in general. There are typically two methods that are given for establishing rights. One is to look at the consequences of letting somebody do something. This is a utilitarian approach which says that the outcomes outweigh any other considerations. So, if the outcomes are really good, then the choice that led to them was a good choice. The utilitarian approach focuses on the actions and their likely outcomes. Our concern is more about the agent performing the decision. If we let so-and-so make the choice, will that likely lead to good outcomes? Much of the argument against letting patients make their own choices falls under this ethical category. The theory is that the physician will pick choices that will lead to better outcomes.

The other option is a rights-based approach, sometimes called the deontological approach. We're going to make this long philosophical story short right here. In the rights-based approach, the consequences do not play a role in establishing rights. A good illustration of this is Judge Cardozo's statement. It refers instead to two features or characteristics that the patient must have to have the right. In this case, the two features are to be an adult and have a sound mind. If you have these, then you are in.

The sound mind acts upon information that is brought in. The informed consent model has a one-way street for that information. It leaves open the question as to why a mind must be sound. How do you judge a mind to be sound? Why in heaven's name are children excluded? In what follows, we try to address these questions.

Continued Significance of Slater

Slater establishes that information is needed for someone to be able to direct what they want or do not want. That is, if we changed up the situation slightly and told Slater what we were going to do, then it would not feel quite so odd. Slater may have had a chance to say, "I really do not want that." Likewise, in the diner, the server could have said, "I'm about to smash this apple pie down your throat," and you could have said, "à la mode?" As preposterous as these examples are, we are reminded that such violations occurred! It becomes clear that information is necessary to have any measure of control over your future, although it may not be sufficient. Without it, you do not have any control. With it, you may have power. There may be some other conditions that are needed to be empowered, as we shall see.

There are at least three items we need to account for in what follows. We need to figure out what a sound mind is, why people think that adults have the right but not children, and finally, how does information play a role between the sound mind and the right to make the choice? Which ethical route you take, the consequentialist or the deontological, will play a substantial role in how you think about these things. However, it's very important to keep in mind that the way we feel about these situations is very strong. The strength of those feelings is not necessarily connected to rational thought.

On we go to the information that is required. We'll return to the diner, as its Yelp scores seem to have increased. Let's see why that might be.

Salgo Hold the Info

Since our last experience at the Paradigm Diner was rather distasteful, maybe we should give it another shot prior to giving our rating on Yelp. We arrive as before. I ask if the waitstaff is the same as last time and am pleasantly surprised to find out that our prior server has since parted ways with the Paradigm Diner. Once seated, we look at the menu. It has three items listed:

Stella's Streetcar	$11.99
Godot's Wait staff Special	$12.99
Gordian's Knot	$8.99

29

This is certainly a bit better. I know prices, but other than the fact that I have three possibilities, you cannot really say much else. It does not appear to be helpful. It is akin to being told that you will have a procedure such as a lithotripsy. Now you may not know what a lithotripsy encapsulates. You have never heard the word before. This goes to the heart of one of the major complaints about physician communication to patients in that it is/was too technical. Physicians were lax in putting things in lay terms.

This dining experience feels a little better than our first visit. At least some respect is being shown, and one cannot say there was no attempt to inform. At least there is no forcing the issue without waiting for the customer. Still, it is unhelpful in making a choice. I would not feel that I controlled the situation. Not enough detail for some diners.

A similar attempt at giving information that was not useful appears in the legal case below. The court finally agrees that you need the information to be autonomous in this context.

Salgo v. Stanford

The case of Salgo v. Leland Stanford Jr. University Board of Trustees is one of the first cases that focuses on the informing piece of the consent process. But better to start at the beginning of the case. Martin Salgo was not a healthy man. Dr. Gerbode was a surgeon employed by Stanford University. He was a well-respected surgeon and a surgery professor at Stanford Medical School.

Martin had a history of an eye condition that indicated premature aging. He was 55. He had started to develop cramping in his legs when walking a few years prior to the events that led to the lawsuit. His physician tried to treat him with medications for about a year. This did not work, so he was referred to Dr. Gerbode, who specialized in treating arterial diseases. His chief complaint at that time was cramping in his legs. It was severe enough to make him limp. The condition had begun earlier and had gradually worsened to the point that his hips and lower back hurt whenever he exercised.

When Gerbode examined Salgo, he noted that Salgo looked much older than his stated age. Both legs appeared atrophied, and his right leg was blue.

When he lifted his legs, they blanched. Based on these physical findings, Dr. Gerbode diagnosed a probable occlusion of the abdominal aorta. In layperson's terms, he had very little blood supply to his legs, and something was blocking his circulation. What Dr. Gerbode could not tell was where the blockage was located or the nature of the blockage. Dr. Gerbode testified that Mr. Salgo had a serious condition.

The next part is telling, and we should remember what the patient and his family are going through at this point. Mr. Salgo has been physically debilitated for quite some time. He is suffering from pain and reduced mobility. Now he is facing the prospect of a frightening diagnosis, although his condition may have forewarned him of this possibility.

Now the language used in the court case may not have been verbatim of what Dr. Gerbode said. However, he could not remember what he told the patient to gain his consent. So, for our purposes, let us assume this is close to what he said. He did tell Salgo that he should go to the hospital for a thorough evaluation. Mr. Salgo needed a study of his aorta, which would involve an anesthetic and the injection of a material into the aorta to localize the blockage. He further elaborated that if the tests confirmed his exam, an operation would improve Mr. Salgo's condition to remove the blockage by removing and replacing a segment of his aorta. "Such an operation would improve the circulation to the legs and back and prolong his life" (Salgo 6 of 20). Dr. Gerbode did not inform Mr. Salgo about any details surrounding the procedures.

Mr. Salgo entered the hospital. He went through a barium swallow, and X-rays were taken from his chest and abdomen. The x-rays showed a marked "calcification in the abdominal aorta, iliac, and femoral vessels" (Salgo 6 of 20). Based on this, Gerbode ordered the aortography through the hospital's person-ray department. Dr. Ellis, a surgeon, would be in charge of this phase of Salgo's stay. An aortography involves inserting a needle into the aorta to inject a radio-opaque substance. The patient lies face down on the table and is anesthetized. While under, the surgeon will insert the needle into the aorta, which lies in front of the spinal column. Based on the testimony, Dr. Ellis had no problems inserting the needle. The injection only took a few seconds.

They took the person's rays and reviewed them while Salgo remained under anesthesia. They decided they needed more pictures and injected more material, though they had left the needle in place. Everything seemed to have gone well. However, when Salgo awoke the next morning, he was paralyzed in his legs. It was a permanent condition.

This was a disaster. It was never determined if there was some negligence on the part of Dr. Ellis slipping the needle through the aorta, or if the needle came out and the material perhaps had leaked into the spinal column. The fact that the procedure led to his paralysis is a tragedy. It is also why a lawsuit was brought in the first case. However, we are here concerned with what Dr. Ellis or Gerbode did or did not inform the family.

The family maintained that neither Drs. Gerbode nor Ellis informed them that something like an aortography would be performed. Both Dr. Gerbode and Dr. Ellis contradicted this. But they added this disclaimer: They admitted that the details of the procedure and the possible dangers were not explained. And there's the rub.

How could this occur? Well, the amount of detail and the nature of the detail necessary to form a decision is highly perspectival. The physicians are already well-versed. They may have even said that they recommended Mr. Salgo undergo an aortography. After all, they know what that means.

Furthermore, they know the risks, but given Mr. Salgo's condition, they may have surmised it was worth the risk. Or they mentioned they would run some tests and take some X-rays. Of course, all of this is true, but the level of detail seems scant at best.

Another interesting factor of this type of disclosure is that it does not seem like a choice to the patient. There is nothing untruthful in what was relayed, but how the situation was portrayed, and the lack of detail made it seem like a foregone conclusion. "You have a serious condition" and "I can add a few more years to your life" sound persuasive, especially when there is nothing on the other side of the ledger to balance it.

The family's background and point of view was most likely quite different. They did not have a medical background. So even if they were told they were going to have an aortography, not describing what it was or the risks involved would not be disclosing enough. Mr. Salgo is not making the decision based on available information. It is straightforward to evaluate this case since the doctors admitted that they did not reveal any risks to the procedure. Zero is not enough.

The practical question, though, is what enough information is, and what is relevant for each patient to support them in their decision-making.

Significance of Salgo: A Court Waffle

There are two thoughts I wish to draw from this case. One is that consent is not enough. In fact, you can say that without an explanation of the meaning of "aortography," no consent was given for the procedure. Information about the intervention itself is clearly required to obtain valid consent. I am not sure you need to consult with the patient to know that you should explain what you intend to do. In Salgo, both parties agreed that the procedure's risks were not divulged, and the court held that besides explaining the nature of the intervention, you also must disclose the risks involved. As for what risks need to be disclosed, the court mentioned "…any facts which are necessary to form the basis of an intelligent consent by the patient to the proposed treatment" (Salgo pp 18-20). This is reasonable but does not offer much practical guidance. The court was struggling with how much information to give to the patient. Their reluctance seems to have been guided by the fear of injuring patients by giving them too much information. They cautioned against giving patients information regarding all the risks, regardless of how remote, since they may result in causing alarm. There are reasons to be concerned with information overload, but the court's reasoning betrays a paternalistic attitude. A patient may refuse treatment because the risk of information overload promotes too much anxiety. This anxiety may interfere with the ability to think things through. That is a risk and a challenge to be met. The court was concerned with a separate set of risks, however. They noted that the fear itself might cause physical harm.

Even allowing for exceptions, information causing physical harm is not something that happens often. There are several good reasons to limit the amount of information given to anyone, not the least of which is that the overload scenario makes it harder to assimilate any of the information. That difficulty is not related to the issue that the court cited. There are enough studies out there that point to the difficulty humans have in processing a lot of information (Kahneman 39 of 570). To complicate it even more, giving a lot of negative information creates a bias around the prospects regardless of the improbabilities of these risks becoming realities. A lot of improbable negative outcomes get overemphasized in the decision process. It creates a gloomy picture.

This back and forth by the court about the risks experienced captures well the difficulties we have coming to grips with decisions about how much and what information to divulge. It is all well and good to divulge all the information that the patient needs to make the decision. But it provides no guidance as to how to figure that out. As a health care provider, am I to guess, as in *Jeopardy*? "I will take Joe's preferences for $400"?

It would clearly help to understand better what concerns are relevant for any individual patient. If the patient participated, it would make this easier, no doubt. More of this later.

The court admonishes us that too much information may be alarming. We know this can be true by looking at behavioral economic studies. Patients may interpret the abundance of information as "Whoa, this must really be bad." The risk could be quite tangential. The court's concern was scaring patients to the point that fright would cause some direct harm, though the court is somewhat vague about the nature of the harm. Would it cause emotional distress, or would it harm the patient's decision-making prowess?

The courts display a lot of waffling between the need to give information and not scaring the living daylights out of the patient. You must "tell them everything they need to know to make a decision" but "don't tell them too much, so they are hurt by the information." Needless to say, but I will say it anyway, this approach really is not helpful. It lacks the guidance necessary to get the right behavior. The challenge to date is that we will try to hit the sweet spot of how much information to give, how to give it, and how to support autonomy and good decisions. Salgo does not hit the mark either, but it is a step forward in protecting autonomy. Moving on...

34

Natanson Diner

After letting the diner owners know you are having trouble selecting, you ask for more details of the choices on the menu. They comply by issuing yet another version of the menu. It now looks like this:

Stella's Streetcar: $11.99
The most desired item on our menu. A delicious blend of roast beef with a wonderful glaze combined with our spice blend. Accompanied by mixed vegetables.

Gordian's Knot: $12.99
A soft pretzel made by hand with our organic dough stuffed with our cheese blend.

Godot's Waitstaff Special: $8.99
A vegan's delight. A green pepper stuffed with rice and vegetables. All topped with our sublime tomato sauce.

This is much better. I have some idea of what I might be tasting and putting into my body. I can make a choice based on this added information. If I am vegan, I know what I can have and what I cannot. I also have a better idea of how Stella's Streetcar might taste. It is possible to imagine what each item tastes like to some extent. Like the nature of an intervention, we kind of know what will happen. But is this enough? Suppose I have various food allergies. Gordian's knot gives me sufficient information to avoid it if I am lactose and/or gluten intolerant. The other two items do not give sufficient information. How detailed should we be when disseminating information to a patient? Certainly, the information is much better, and one is more likely to make a good choice than before. But it is still possible to select the wrong item for you given your tastes and situation. It might not be disastrous for most of us, no matter what we select, so we would be okay with any choices. It helps the lactose intolerant. But the spiced item may be too spicy. There may be unspecified ingredients in the dishes that pose a danger to some people. Some people can go into anaphylactic shock when exposed to nuts or even certain spices. Some will already know they are allergic, but others will not, with the latter forming a particular difficulty.

Natanson and Risk

The challenge of specificity of information is a challenging one. Take the case of Natanson v Kline. This brings up an interesting departure from our one-way model of information flow from physician to the patient. How much information is relevant to making a choice with the HCP (or waitstaff), and how much is with the patient (patron)? The issue is that patients must be informed about risks to the degree relevant to their patient's values. How is the HCP supposed to know what the patient values or prefers? Initially, the courts managed this by resorting to what any rational patient would deem relevant. Frankly, it really was left up to a jury to decide what was relevant. Let us look at the following court case of Natanson v Kline.

Imagine being Irma Natanson. You have just had surgery which has significantly altered your appearance. You are aware you have just dodged a bullet. Yet things seem to be going well. Your surgeon has made a recommendation to see a radiologist. At this point, it would be natural for Irma to trust Dr. Crumpacker. The trust built up by Dr. Crumpacker would naturally extend over to his recommendation of Dr. Kline and cobalt therapy.

Irma Natanson was suffering from breast cancer. She had a left mastectomy performed by Dr. Crumpacker. He determined that she needed radiation therapy as a follow-up. He referred her to Dr. Kline. Based on Dr. Crumpacker's suggestion, the Natansons sought out Dr. Kline. He felt that cobalt was the treatment of choice. Now cobalt is a radioactive substance and, at the time of this proposed intervention (circa 1960), had not been used. There was not much experience with it. In fact, the protocol required having a physicist attend the administration of the product. In hindsight, this is a real warning signal when the team needs to include a nuclear physicist.

Unfortunately, the patient was given a dose that for her was too high. As a result, Irma had an ulcer under her left arm (the size of a quarter) from the mastectomy and testified that she thought the radiation treatment was supposed to help close it up. To her chagrin, it drained even more and seemed to grow larger. In the summary given as part of the instructions to the original jury, the instruction stated: "that Dr. Kline and personnel of Francis Hospital administered to the plaintiff a series of cobalt radiation treatments in such a manner that the skin, flesh, and muscles beneath her left arms sloughed away and ribs of her left chest were so burned that they became necrotic or dead" (Natanson 8 of 26). So, this is what Irma Natanson had suffered through. That is not to say the doctors had necessarily behaved negligently.

The court case itself was mostly based on the idea that the doctors were negligent in treating her. That, in fact, they had given her too high a dosage. There was plenty of conflicting testimony around this, and the jury returned in favor of the doctors. The Natansons were appealing the case based on the notion that the doctors were negligent as a matter of law, not facts. What this means is that some facts that were not disputed in the testimony were tantamount to negligence.

It is interesting to note that in discussing the lower court proceedings, the appellate court included reflections on the part of the physicians that they "had taken a calculated risk"in providing the treatment (Natanson 7 of 26). Now we do not have access to the original court testimony, but there certainly are calculated risks to any intervention. The question before us is who should be doing the calculating, because the phrasing belies the bias. "The physicians took a calculated risk." Really? The patient takes the risks. The patient could not have taken a calculated risk without knowing the risk. This risk of injury was never communicated to her. She had nothing to calculate.

Natanson lost at trial and appealed the ruling. Much of the appeal (and this is true of appeals) concerned technical legal issues. However, it was born out in the testimony that the procedure's risks were never detailed to her by the staff. At most, the Natansons were told that this treatment was like any other and, as such, had risks associated with it. In fact, part of the doctor's testimony was that he had to use an extremely high dose, one right on the edge of safety. This fact should have been communicated to the patient.

One of Natanson's allegations was that Dr. Kline did not disclose that the intended treatment involved a great risk of bodily injury or death. They had wanted the court to instruct the jury in the following words:

> "You are instructed that the relationship between physician and patient is a fiduciary one. The relationship requires the physician to make a full disclosure to the patient of all matters within his knowledge affecting the interests of the patient. Included within the matters which the physician must advise the patient are the nature of the proposed treatment and any hazards of the proposed treatment which are known to the physician. Every adult person has the right to determine for himself or herself whether or not he will subject his body to hazards of any particular medical treatment. You are instructed that if you find from the evidence that defendant Kline knew that the treatment, he proposed to administer to plaintiff involved hazards or danger he was under a duty to advise plaintiff of that fact and if you further find that defendant Kline did not advise plaintiff of such hazards then defendant Kline was guilty of negligence." (10 of 26)

This is quite a mouthful. The appellate court was grappling with the issue of how to instruct a jury sufficiently without biasing them. The appellate court clearly connects the information regarding risks and valid consent. "We are here concerned with a case where the patient consented to the treatment but alleges in a malpractice action that the nature and consequences of the risks of the treatment were not properly explained to her. This relates directly to the question whether the physician has obtained the informed consent of the patient to render the treatment administered" (3 Of 26). What details of the risks should have been transmitted in this case?

The technical details of cobalt radiation were detailed in court testimony by Dr. Kline. Facts such as how powerful the radiation is and that many feet of concrete are required to house the machine indicate that the procedure is inherently dangerous. The controls are operated in an adjoining room which is monitored periodically for any increases in radiation there. As pointed out by the appellate court, these sorts of facts are not commonly known, and as such, patients cannot be expected to know the hazards of radiation treatment using radioactive cobalt. They would need to have the radiologist inform them. "While Dr. Kline did not testify that the radiation he gave the appellant (Irma) caused her injury, he did state cobalt irradiation could cause the injury which the appellant did sustain" (13 of 26).

The court asks itself one of the questions we are asking. "What is the extent of a physician's duty to confide in his patient where the physician suggests or recommends a particular treatment? What duty is there upon him to explain the nature and the probable consequences of that treatment to the patient? To what extent should he disclose the existence and nature of the risks inherent in the treatment?" (13 of 26). At the end of the day, the court proclaimed that physicians should divulge what other physicians divulge in like circumstances. A bit unfulfilling, I would say. I mean, that would leave it open to divulging little if physicians commonly do it.

The court, rightly, I believe, goes on to review other cases where although there is a clear duty to disclose, it does not seem warranted that a physician is obligated to disclose every detail. Considering all the possible details and paths of consequences, it can be impractical to relay every potential known adverse effect from treatment. So, we are left with the challenge of providing the right amount of detail.

Significance of Natanson

Natanson shows an improvement over Salgo. The information is general, and the degree of danger was never transmitted to Natanson. Like the diner example, you can better understand what you will be getting into. You were told the procedure was not risk-free. You also know you are getting radiation. In either the diner case or the legal one, you do not know how much risk you are exposed to or the details of the diner food or the radiation intervention. So let us try to remedy the situation.

Canterbury Diner Tales

Our next turn at the Paradigm Diner offers a bit more. The menu this time looks like this:

Stella's Streetcar: $11.99
The most desired item on our menu. A delicious blend of roast beef with a wonderful glaze combined with our spice blend of cumin, oregano, and cayenne pepper, accompanied by mixed vegetables.

Gordian's Knot: $12.99
A soft pretzel made by hand with our organic dough stuffed with our own cheese blend.

Godot's Wait staff Special: $8.99
A vegan's delight. A green pepper stuffed with basmati rice and sauteed in olive oil, green peppers, and onions. All topped with the usual sauce.

Canterbury's Tale

A few more morsels for our gustatory consideration.

This next case probes a bit further (Canterbury v Spence). The story began when Jerry Canterbury was 19. He experienced pain between his shoulder blades. He sought out two different physicians, but their prescriptions did not offer enough relief. Canterbury got an appointment with a neurosurgeon, Dr. Spence. A laminectomy (removing the part of the disc impinging on the spinal nerves) was going to be required. However, Dr. Spence discovered several anomalies upon getting into the spinal column. He relieved a lot of the pressure on the spinal cord by enlarging the outer protective wall.

On the first day, post-op, Canterbury was progressing normally. At some point, he felt the need to urinate. Dr. Spence had left orders that Canterbury should remain in bed while voiding. Someone changed the orders so that voiding could be done out of bed. Canterbury called for the nurse and was given the urine bottle, but was left unattended. He managed a scenario between both sets of orders. He slipped off the side of the bed and fell to the floor.

A few hours later, he complained that he could not move his legs and he was having trouble breathing. Dr. Spence was notified, and Mrs. Canterbury was rushed to the hospital. Canterbury's mother signed another consent form, and the young Canterbury was taken to the operating room. Spence created more room for his spinal cord.

His muscles improved somewhat after a second operation, but he still had trouble voiding and paralysis of his bowels. By the time of the appeal, he was still suffering from these medical problems. As if this were not enough, he could not hold a job because he was always seated and needed to be close to a bathroom.

There are many issues here, but our concern is what Dr. Spence disclosed to the Canterbury family about the operation. The court noted that physicians have a "responsibility of satisfying the vital information needs of the patient. More recently, we have found in the fiducial qualities of the physician-patient relationship the physician's duty to reveal to the patient that which is in his best interests it is important that he should know." "We now find, as part of the physician's overall obligation to the patient, a similar duty of reasonable disclosure of the choices with respect to proposed therapy and the dangers, inherently and potentially involved." (Canterbury para. 31).

This last sentence clearly states that the disclosure (for legal purposes) involves the dangers immediate to the therapy and those that could potentially occur. The court pointed out that for the consent to be valid, informed consent must disclose the options and perils of the therapies.

But in the law and in practice, the HCP faces the daunting task of how much detail to provide. None is too little, and everything they understand about each option is too much. That would require the patient to go through medical training. The court struggled with defining the line between adequate and non-adequate disclosure. So shall we. In this case, we can see that the surgeon understood the danger of falling, which is why he wanted the patient to remain on bedrest.

At the time, different standards were used in the courts to evaluate whether enough information was disclosed. On the one side was the professional standard. That would be the case where the typical disclosure by physicians would be the standard. On the other side of the ledger would be what the patient requires. The latter approach is in concert with what we see here from an ethical point of view. It means that the staff needs to communicate in a way that is tailored to the particular patient. In the case of the Canterbury appellate court, they opined that the "test for determining whether a particular peril must be divulged is its materiality to the patient's decision: all risks potentially affecting the decision must be unmasked."

This sounds great until you consider that unless the physician is a mind reader, they cannot know in advance what or what would not be relevant. Later I will argue that they can come closer and that the patient needs to participate in the discussion. The court took a different tack. They adopted the reasonable person standard. "A risk is thus material when a reasonable person, in what the physician knows or should know to be the patient's position, would be likely to attach significance to the risk or cluster of risks in deciding whether to forego the proposed therapy" (Canterbury para. 44).

At least this pragmatic approach puts more of an obligation on the HCP to divulge risks they think reasonable people would want to know. In this case, the risk of paralysis seems like something I would want to know, or any reasonable person would want to know. The court went on to articulate that the disclosure needs to include items that may be of less probability, but of such significance that a prudent person would want to be aware of them.

Our purpose is not so much to have any change in the legal approach to these matters. We want to reach a better practice in the medical context rather than legal remedies—at least in the context of this book. There are two exceptions to the legal rule.

First, there is no duty to disclose when patients cannot consent (say they are unconscious). The second exception to the duty to disclose is when risk disclosure poses a threat of detriment to the patient. The hypothesis is that disclosing information may make the patient so upset that they would not be able to make a rational decision.

Now here is something for us. The idea is to make it possible for the patient to make the best decision. At some point, one must place some responsibility on the patient. The court was quite aware that this latter exception could ultimately lead to permanently voiding the patient's right to ultimately choose if it is not the one that the HCP thinks is the best.

The court also addressed the issue of evaluating whether a certain risk should have been divulged to the patient. The court rejected the notion of using the test of whether the patient would have chosen differently. They point out a legitimate issue in actual cases. The cases are brought forward because the risk was realized. This creates a bias in the decision-making post facto that cannot be overcome.

So, the court opted for a different method of evaluation. This method can assist the HCP in informing the patient what items to reveal. The court offered the prudent person standard. In other words, what would a prudent person in the patient's position have decided if suitably informed of all perils bearing significance? In other words, would a reasonable person have declined the treatment if there had been adequate disclosure?

This appeals court has broken with the tradition of the evaluation of treating disclosure of information similarly to any other medical procedure. This would leave the standard to be irrevocably attached to the medical practice. If most physicians did not disclose the risk of paralysis, Canterbury would be out of luck.

For our purposes, we wish to go a step further than the courts. We are not so concerned with practical legal matters. Our concern is with doing what we can to bring about the best circumstances for patients. In so doing, we can provide useful suggestions that could be incorporated into legal considerations. Our view is that the divide between the physician and the patient is not the best model. There are better models than the divide between the physician and the patient. They take the position that the problem has been poorly articulated and that it creates an unnecessary divide. The historical approach articulated by these courts treats the situation as one where the physician is simply transmitting data to the patient, rather than seeing it as a social situation involving communication.

Well, so much for the principles of the case. So, what did Dr. Spence disclose regarding the laminectomy? According to Mr. Canterbury, Dr. Spence did not say anything about any hazards associated with the surgery. Canterbury's mother testified that she asked (notice that Spence did not offer) about the dangers of the laminectomy. He responded that it was no more dangerous than any other surgery. Let us perform our procedure on that type of response because it is instructive in many ways.

Significance of Canterbury

There are two people here, both with their own set of beliefs and backgrounds. Mind you, Dr. Spence intentionally did not disclose the hazards because he believed the information would have led the patient to decline the surgery. This is interesting on several grounds. The first is that the information would so distress the patient that he could not think straight. If true, that might be a morally significant piece of data and would lead the doctor to not inform the patient. After all, one could argue that the patient was rendered incompetent by the information. Once incompetent, the right to make the decision might pass to someone else.

It could be that the doctor wants to achieve the best possible outcome. Even though the patient may most likely agree to go ahead and the good doctor thinks that way, the doctor believes that the information will make the patient pessimistic about the outcome of the intervention, which in turn will lead to a worse outcome.

This is the very height of a paternalistic point of view. Patients are not responsible for their actions. They are children. So even if the physician is correct that the outcomes might be worse, it is upon the patient to rectify.

During my nursing career, I encountered numerous patients who preferred not to think these things through. Typical responses to the situation would be, "Doctor, just do what you think is best." This could have been motivated by numerous factors. The stress of the situation might have made the decision one more thing to bear. Or it could be that they did not want to have to translate what they were being told in any meaningful way. It could have been both.

The statement that the laminectomy had similar dangers as any other surgery is false. It is the case that it shares with other surgeries the risks associated with anesthesia. However, it also risks paralysis of the lower limbs, bowel, and bladder function. That danger to the patient is not shared with, say, an appendectomy. This sort of cavalier approach to the meaning of the risks creates a road to failure in communication. It is natural to project our understanding onto others. It is also natural to project our own experience into the situation. In Dr. Spence's defense here, it is possible that the terrible sequelae had nothing to do with him. In fact, it really was not the surgery itself that went bad. He even left proper instructions not to let Canterbury out of bed. It must be admitted, though, that had Canterbury been fortified with the risk of paralysis given a fall post-surgery, he might never have attempted to sit up unattended.

What would Mrs. Canterbury have thought at the time? Dr. Spence was downplaying the risks even to her. It appears the very act of suppressing other risks makes them take on more importance and relevance to the situation. However, it is possible, and we do not know because we were not there, that he thought the risk was so remote that it was not worth divulging. Regardless of what the actual Dr. Spence thought, we now know there is a relevance to this line of thinking in light of studies in behavioral economics. By divulging a lot of important and highly imaged possibilities, we tend to place a higher belief in their probability than is warranted. Repetition of risks makes it seem like they are more prevalent (Kahneman 89 of 570).

The impetus to do good is prevalent in medicine. It is one of the primary motivators for people to undertake the profession. Knowing what a patient needs to be informed of is incredibly challenging. The situation is typically one where the stakeholders are strangers. If we wish to make this work under stressful circumstances, then we can maximize the best outcome if both parties understand that they have to communicate. And the emphasis on *both parties* is essential. The stakeholders do not have an equal footing in this, as the physician is typically in the "stronger" position. The standard view is that the physician possesses the information the patient needs to make a proper choice. Since the choice belongs to the patient, the physician needs nothing from the patient. But there is a hole in this version. If the physician is under some moral obligation to help the patient, they also need information from the patient.

The patient also needs to be on the hook here.

Now in the case of Canterbury, all parties most likely understand the outcome of a paralysis and permanent incontinence. But the difficulty here is that the proximal cause of the event was not the surgery itself. Spence could have informed Canterbury that the surgery itself had a chance of causing these issues directly without the fall. And the fact that the fall was caused proximally by slipping off the bed, which may have been the result of the surgery, is unknown. Assuming it is, then the warning to the patient and the staff not to let him up means that Spence was cognizant of the fact that this was a known risk of the surgery. In other words, if the patient fell after surgery, the patient stood at a greater risk of paralysis than if he had fallen prior to the surgery. Alternatively, Spence may have known that the patient was more likely to have a fall post-surgery than before and that he was likely to have an injury with or without the surgery. The fact that Spence instructed the staff that he was on bedrest and not to get up unassisted is appropriate. That he did not warn the patient of the information is not.

But why this dichotomy? Why is it either hand over information or keep it close to the vest? Why do we not have the option of supporting the patient through the choice, helping them assess the alternatives, and as much as possible, letting them work their way through the process? But I contend that the patient has an obligation to make the decision if competent. The longer we keep the patient passive, the harder it is to meet the goals.

Diner Cobbs

Stella's Streetcar: $11.99
The most desired item on our menu. A delicious blend of roast beef with a wonderful glaze combined with our spice blend of cumin, oregano, and cayenne pepper and accompanied by mixed vegetables.

Gordian's Knot: $12.99
A soft pretzel made by hand with our organic dough stuffed with our cheese blend.

Godot's Wait staff Special: $8.99
A vegan's delight. Green pepper stuffed with basmati rice and sauteed in olive oil, green peppers, and onions. All topped with our sublime tomato sauce.

The Godot's Wait staff special looked good, and one of my colleagues ordered it on the advice of our server. Within five minutes, they exhibited signs of a reaction. Extreme nausea ensued. We asked the server what was in the sauce, and it turned out it contained almonds. It would have been good to know. Reducing information to guide the customer is contrary to letting the customer decide.

Cobbs v Grant

This case involves Ralph Cobbs, who was suffering from a duodenal ulcer. He was admitted to the hospital in 1964. He underwent tests to measure the severity of the condition. He was treated with oral medication but continued to suffer and complained of lower abdominal pain and nausea. Cobbs was being attended to by Dr. Jerome Sands, his family physician. Dr. Sands felt that surgery was indicated. At this point, Sands explained to the patient, in general terms, the risks of receiving a general anesthetic. Dr. Sands called in a surgeon Dr. Dudley F.P. Grant. Grant examined Cobbs and concluded that the patient had an intractable peptic duodenal ulcer, which would require surgery. Dr. Grant explained the nature of the surgery. What was missing in the conversation? No discussion of risks. So, at this point, Cobbs was given information about the procedure and the risks associated with getting the general anesthetic.

The surgery took place the day after the consent, and it appeared to have gone extremely well. The ulcer was gone. Eight days later, Cobbs was permitted to go home as he progressed nicely. The day after he went home, Cobbs began to experience intense pain in his abdomen. He called up Dr. Sands, who had him admitted to the hospital. Two hours after readmission, Cobbs went into shock. Emergency surgery was performed. He was internally bleeding due to a severed artery at the hilum of the spleen. Dr. Grant decided to remove the spleen, as it is not necessary to have a spleen as an adult. It turns out that the original procedure to repair the ulcer has a noted risk of injuries to the spleen. In fact, it happens in about 5 percent of the cases. As has been stated, this risk had not been disclosed.

Cobbs' unfortunate saga continued. He recuperated for two weeks in the hospital. Guess what happened a month after he had returned home? Yup, you guessed it. He had sharp pains in his stomach and was readmitted. Tests showed that he now had a gastric ulcer. Generating a new ulcer is a risk when you have surgery on an existing duodenal ulcer, which of course, started this cascade of events. The physicians tried to treat the gastric ulcer conservatively with antacids and diet, which were available then. Just to finish the case off and prior to Cobbs suffering any demise, they had to remove 50 percent of his stomach to reduce its acid production. Once again, he was discharged but had to return for an internal bleed caused by the premature absorption of a suture, another risk of surgery. A risk that could have been disclosed.

Significance of Cobbs

The court spelled out four postulates very nicely surrounding informed consent. I will summarize the points.

1. Most patients are not educated in the medical sciences. Consequently, the courts can assume that there is a disparity between the knowledge of the patient and the physician.
2. Any person of adult years and sound mind has the right to control their own body in so far as to determine whether or not to submit to treatment.
3. Patient consent to treatment must be an informed consent. Otherwise, the consent is not effective.
4. "…the patient, being unlearned in medical sciences, has an abject dependence upon and trust in his physician for the information upon which he relies during the decisional process, thus raising an obligation in the physician that transcends arms-length transactions." (Cobbs 17)

The court concluded that it is necessary for a physician to divulge all the information relevant to a meaningful decisional process. "It is the prerogative of the patient, not the physician, to determine for himself the direction in which he believes his interests lie." (Cobbs 18)

The court wrestled with the disclosure issue and what would be relevant. However, they noted that the judgment to be made was a non-medical one. The physician's obligation ends when they describe the risks of treatment or non-treatment and the probability of a successful outcome from the treatment. "The weighing of these risks against the individual subjective fears and hopes of the patient is not an expert skill. Such evaluation and decision are a nonmedical judgment" (Cobbs 20).

Okay, so how much needs to be disclosed by the physician? The court took a stab at it. First, they criticized full disclosure. The need for a polysyllabic lecture is not the goal of this social activity. Nor should doctors need to describe the minor risks of low incidence, which are commonly known to be included in a common procedure. I am still determining what those are. However, the complicated procedure in the Cobbs case did not fall under this notion of a common and simple procedure, so the physicians had a duty to inform Cobb of the risks.

All in all, the court seems to be trying to have it both ways. The doctor must tell the patient the important risks, but not everything, and what is important is what, after the fact, is discovered. The practical piece is that the court set a minimum standard of at least what a competent patient needs to know to make a rational decision.

In summary, the court did make some progress in that they have finally switched over to the fact that the patient makes the decision, and it needs to be based on the patient's fears and hopes. Similarly, our menu choice is somewhat dependent on understanding risks, which is not to be minimized based on what the server prefers or their judgment about risks worth taking. On the other hand, there is still no real patient participation in the information exchange process before the decision. Consequently, when approaching which risks to disclose, they will resort to a standard that is not specific to me. The doctor does not know me. Maybe the health care provider should ask.

Chapter 3

Decision-Making Model: Shift the Paradigm

Gambling

Historically the move toward decision-making models from certainty to uncertainty began in the 17th century. One of the first people to articulate such a theory was Blaise Pascal, the 17th-century mathematician and philosopher. The same idea was voiced independently by Pierre de Fermat, though the two had correspondence on the matter. Pascal was at the forefront of breaking away from how one would come to believe in something. This period in European history was one of transitioning from the scholastic theology governing the times. Science was on the upsurge with thinkers like Descartes, Leibniz, Newton, Spinoza, and Pascal. Pascal and Descartes both helped set the stage for the Enlightenment. At the time of their writing, some figures were beginning to break away from a strict reliance on belief based on the church's authority and scripture.

In some cases, innovative ideas were drawn from observation, but most were grounded in rational thought. Philosophers consider Descartes, Leibniz, and Spinoza the three great Rationalists. These thinkers took great risks as they published works that might seem contrary to church doctrine. It is no wonder that some of their works were published posthumously. On the other hand, most were believers as well. Notably, the three Rationalists believed in God. Rather than resting on biblical text for their proof, they all resorted to rational proofs for God's existence.

The new science was based on observations and reason, and God was not directly observed. Instead, they offered a deductive argument—called the

51

ontological argument—which purported to prove that God existed because the idea of God itself contains the property of existence. One particular version (e.g., Descartes in his Meditations) is that the idea of God includes perfection; if God did not exist, he wouldn't be perfect. Therefore, God must exist. At least in their minds, they were combining their new way of thinking about reality and accommodating their religious beliefs with it. It is difficult breaking away from an old paradigm that you grew up with, even if you're going to be a trailblazer in creating a new one.

Another approach can be found in Blaise Pascal's famous argument. Pascal deviated from this approach significantly. In his *Pensées*, published posthumously in 1670, the choice wouldn't be the result of a deduction but rather in the form of a bet (Pascal section 343). A theological FanDuel if you will. Pascal presented the rationale for a belief in God in the form of a wager recognizing that the ontological argument was /is suspect. He posited that it makes more sense to believe when one weighs the potential outcomes of believing versus not believing.

The argument goes like this:

1. If you choose to believe, then—if correct—you will go to Heaven. A fantastic outcome.
2. If you are wrong—well, what is the harm? Maybe a lot of Sundays are taken up when they otherwise would not. Not a horrible deal.

On the other hand:

3. If you choose not to believe and are right, you get those Sundays back and do not have to follow specific theological rules depending on your faith. In his case, it was Catholicism.
4. If you are wrong, you go to Hell.

For Pascal, the tradeoffs are clear. Even though there are no efforts at placing probabilities on the outcomes, the scenario has come to be known as

Pascal's wager. This brings up another crucial element that will be required of our decision-making model. Whatever we choose, values must be able to be combined in a consistent fashion. Possible gains need to be compared to possible losses to sum things up.

What is of primary importance for us is that Pascal is setting up a situation that involves a rather important choice to make when you don't buy into the certainty of a deductive argument. You might know the J. S. Mill version: "All men are mortal. Socrates is a man. Therefore, Socrates is mortal" (174 of 989). This is known as a valid syllogistic argument in that, given the two premises, the conclusion follows. Once you assume the premises are true, you can deduce the conclusion and be certain about it. Once you introduce uncertainty and probabilities, then you require a different model for rational decision-making. Pascal is arguing to make a choice based on the value of the outcomes to people. This is the basis for any utilitarian approach and illustrates that the potential outcomes need to be assessed within the decision so that they may be compared one against the other.

Gambling scenarios are made for this task. The outcomes to be compared are in currency. The expected value of any gamble is the probability of the outcome times the pot. It does not depend in any way on the wealth of the gamblers or how much that pot will mean to them.

Bernoulli recognized that people do not feel the same about probabilities as the expected value theory dictates. The Saint Petersburg paradox led him to the conclusion that we were more inclined to measure things around net gains and losses than absolute gains and losses. The simple illustration of the problem goes as follows: you are presented with the choice of making a wager with your marbles. Let's make the total number of marbles one thousand. All are blue except for one, which is red. The payoff will be $100. You can wager the $1 to win the $100. We already know that the expected value will be well below $1. From a rational point of view, you should not bet. However, it doesn't seem all that outlandish to go ahead and place the bet because, after all, it is only one dollar. This is similar to how people approach national lotteries. The odds of winning are astronomically bad. But if you throw a couple of bucks into the hopper, it is as if the loss of those two dollars doesn't have the same value as winnings dollars would. We'll see in a lot of behavioral economics studies that most people respond to these choice situations similarly. There's a utility associated with the value of the outcome that is different from the value of the outcome. If I lose a dollar, it is no big deal. Winning one hundred is kind of a big deal. Suppose I lose $2 on the lottery again, no big deal. If I went and bought 50,000 tickets and spent $100,000, then we are talking significant cash and a major negative impact on my happiness if I lose. I will use my very simple P*V equals expected value in all these cases. Yet clearly, there are two senses of the word value in these circumstances. The first is the dollar amount, and the other is what those dollars mean to me in particular.

We begin to see the divergence between the standard model for rational decision-making with uncertainties and risks versus how we think. From a purely monetary point of view, a dollar is a dollar is a dollar. My utilitarian point of view is that not all dollars are alike, especially when they decide to gather together in a larger pool.

Another way to regard this is to think about how much money might mean to a poverty-stricken person compared to a wealthy billionaire. Somebody having trouble making ends meet will find $100 "more valuable" than a multibillionaire who may look at it as a rounding error. In other words, in one case, it may be life-changing and, in the other case, have no impact at all.

Better examples in terms of our intuitions are when we pit certainty against the uncertainty on which Kahneman and Tversky focused their attention (Tversky s258-s261). Suppose I had a chance to place a wager where I was guaranteed $48 or a 50 percent chance of winning $100. Most people would take the $48 though that has a lower expected value. (0.50 *100) = an EV of $50. This type of problem choice led Bernoulli to the notion of marginal utilities. These utilities are based on the change in value for someone rather than some absolute number. This certainly is not the end of the story, but it is a very good beginning. Likewise, the changes in value can be gauged against the baseline for the subject. It really places some emphasis on the individual and their own situation: expected values and expected utilities. The expected value is objective and is known without referencing any individual. The utility of that value will differ between us based on our circumstances and makeup. If I am rich (oh, if only I were!), then winning or losing twenty dollars does not offer much utility. If we are talking about a million dollars, then we are talking. If I were destitute, then that dollar may have more utility in that it might sustain me or help sustain me.

The utility of an outcome is important to the types of situations we are encountering here. It does allow us to personalize the outcomes and still remain in the realm of calculation.

The Expected Value (EV) Model

Consider gambles placed for a pot of money. If you win, it will be all the money in the pot. It will not be a fraction of that money. If you have a 20 percent chance of winning $100, then you have an expected value of $.2*$100 = 20. On the other hand, if you win, you get $100.

As you can see, the expected value of an outcome is about probable outcomes. If you run the gamble one hundred times, you will win about 20 times. Run it one thousand times, and you should get the win rate to about 200 times. It is more about how frequently you will win, and so over a period of tries, you get what your expected results will be. Each time you win, you'll get $100.

The EV model works extremely well for outcomes that are mathematical quantities. After all, the algorithm is arithmetical. To perform the arithmetic, you are required to have two numbers. The fact that the formula is a mathematical formula brings some other properties rarely discussed in this context. One of these is incredibly important, though, and it is the notion of precision. This will get overlooked quite easily in gambling scenarios. The currency has its own precision, as does the probability. An example of this is that the most precise estimate for currency is to go two places to the right of the decimal point if you are exchanging dollars. Depending upon the circumstances, the probabilities may have more or less precision (numbers to the right of the decimal point). The math rule is that the product of two numbers can only have the precision of the least precise number. So, if the probability is .2015 and the currency value of the payoff is

$420.02, then the result will need to be rounded to the second decimal place. .2015 * $420.02 = $84.63403. The extra numbers to the right need to be rounded to the least precise numbers to the right of the decimal point from the two multipliers. The second one 420.02 only goes two places to the right of the decimal. That fact will govern how far to the right the product of the two numbers can legitimately go. That would be an expected value of $84.63. This seemingly innocuous arithmetic characteristic turns out to have important consequences.

The question to ask when we are supplying our own values is "how precise can we be?" The EV model requires us to supply a number for the value of the outcome we seek. When I compare my preferences or values, it is not even close to this kind of precision. It is more like the order of magnitude. I am not sure of what steps I take in comparing outcomes. It is rarely a conscious thing with a ton of clarity. I make a ranking without reference to probabilities. For me to take notice, I would need a large disparity of probabilities. This has important implications.

Our context is different from these gambling scenarios. I find it quite fascinating that this is not written about all that much.

Another gambling scenario for the marble example looks like this:
Option 1: Don't play.
Option 2: Make the bet on an outcome.

Now, consider how the context for decision-making in health care might look. We get our first set of options to say they are to operate or take meds.

The options initially look like this:
Option 1: Do nothing.
Option 2: Take medication.
Option 3: Have surgery.

Each option has its own outcomes with its own probabilities.
A tree diagram can represent these choice problems. Another important discovery will be made once we do this.

It is possible to use a visual approach to illustrate decisions like this. It is called a tree diagram. Here is the $2 bet on pulling out the red marble from the jug which contains one red and 9 blue marbles.

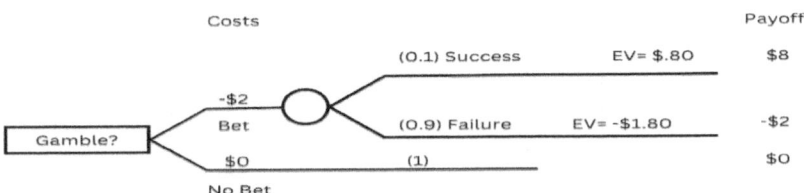

Figure 1 Calculations for choosing to bet or not to bet in the urn problem.

The expected value for the two options needs to be calculated. The don't place a bet option is simply $0*0 + 0*0 = 0$. Not an unexpected result going down the left branch. Let's see what happens going down the right branch. $(.1*\$10) + (.9*\$0) -\$2$. The minus reflects the amount of the bet. The math works out to an EV of - $1. We now compare the results from each choice. Well, the not playing landed on $0, and playing landed on -$1. The result is clear you are better off not playing the game. No more branches or extensions of the tree are needed. There is a certain elegance to this processing. The entire process is quite seductive. It is complete, precise, and will never let you down if you deploy it correctly in gambling-type situations. The real question for us is not whether it works in this area involving numbers (and they are given to us), but if it also will work in the medical context where we have to supply the values in terms of their magnitudes.

Let us expand on the choices for the medical situation. We can use type 2 diabetes as an example. For our purposes here, I have combined some possible oral drugs. Side effects vary greatly, as does efficacy, but in large measure, it appears to be individual. Oral drugs seem to be less effective over time for reasons unknown. They are also less effective for type 2 diabetes.

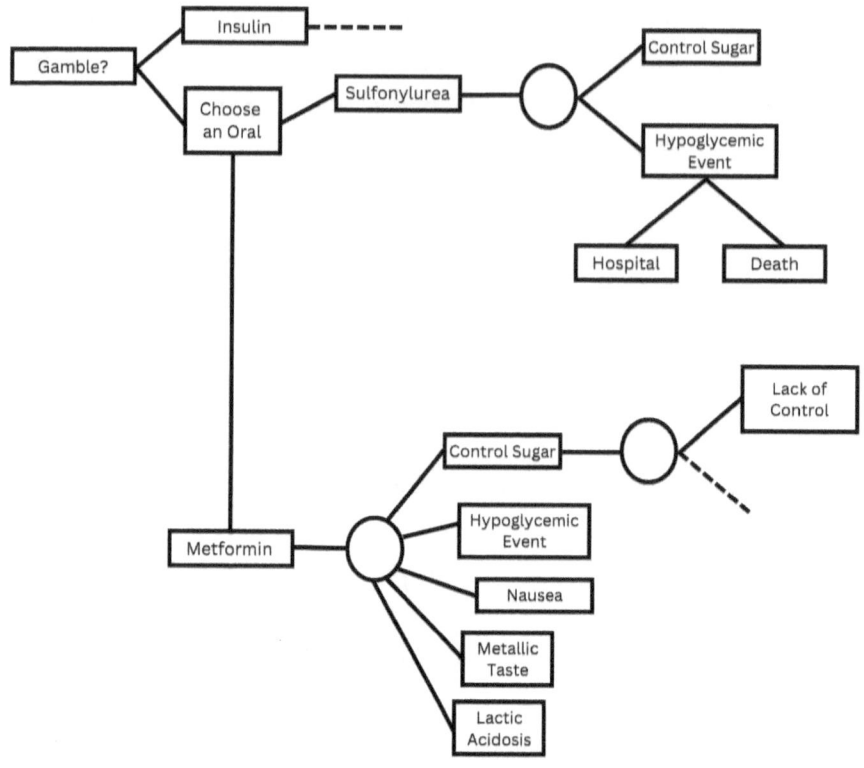

Figure 2 Insulin v Oral Diabetic medication decision trees (truncated)

Let us interrupt Figure 2 at this juncture. We have yet to add the probabilities and values for the various boxes in the decision tree. One difference between this figure and the previous one should be obvious, namely, how much larger it is. In fact, it will extend downwards and out for quite some time, with more probabilities, values, and choices to be entered. You will know that even though there are three alternatives initially, there are at least eight different outcomes to be valued. We are only at the first level at this point. Based on these outcomes, there'll be more to add to the chart. I would suggest that this becomes the most impractical task at this point. The EV model doesn't tell us where to stop. I can imagine that this stems from the use of gambling examples at its very origin. Those problems have a natural ending point: the gamble's outcome.

How far down will it extend? This is a tricky situation. Figure 1 is easy.

The tree ends at the same point regardless of choice. Two of the choices happen at the same moment in time. Figure 2 is a different animal altogether. Some branches will end sooner than others. When do we make the comparisons between the branches? The longer the branches, the more unwieldy the calculations. Even making calculations is problematic. The values in the gambling sample are discreet. They are not continuous values. We would have to convert medical values similarly. This is not to say it can't be done. It is hard to see that this is a theoretical limitation in Figure 2. However, it quickly gets to be impractical. Let us look at trying to create values for illustration purposes.

The fact is that the values in the medical example are more continuous in nature rather than discrete, as in the gambling scenarios. Let us unpack this notion of our outcomes in medicine, as they are more of a continuous variable. (I assume death is probably the most discreet of all those variables.)

One of the potential side effects of, say, metformin is to have some nausea. What is the negative value I place on nausea? Is it related to intensity? Well, is it related to duration? If that is so, is it by minutes, by hour or by day? After all, the math would have us multiply the probability of that outcome times its value. Do we have to sum that value up over a certain duration of time? The model seems to be less enticing than it was before. I suppose one solution to this duration issue is that a person would have to project the duration of the nausea so long as the intensity of it was the same. Once the intensity decreases, presumably, the negative value gets diminished, and there's a new duration for each diminishment. The math is getting more unwieldy by the moment.

Another challenge concerns the placement of a value on an outcome. The value has to be mapped onto an arithmetic scale to stay within this model. We typically do this in health care. One is often asked on a scale of zero to ten how much pain you think you have, with ten being the worst pain you've ever had and zero being no pain at all. Here the degree of precision comes into play in that we're dealing with whole numbers. There is also no guarantee that the scale is linear, meaning that the increase in pain from two to three may not be the same as the increase in pain from eight to nine. There is also no guarantee that I will be consistent with these scales over time. These two challenges don't make it impossible to use the model of expected value in the informed consent paradigm; it just starts losing its elegance quickly in this context. It's so easy to get the probabilities of an intervention's outcomes from an objective database, and it's so easy to get currency that is the same value for all people. A dollar is a dollar is a dollar. But the values in health care are quite subjective in the sense that they are related to a personal perspective.

Problems for the Expected Value Decision-Making Model

Using the EV model in the context of informed consent presents several problems in the model's applicability. For me, the most striking issue is that no one I know or have met thinks this way naturally. If we must choose a decision model, then it is better not to choose an impractical one if something else can be made available. The EV approach doesn't seem to be one likely to be easily implemented. Compliance with this model is difficult. In fact, many of the researchers in Behavioral Economics regard this as the ideal decision model and bemoan the fact that we don't typically deploy the tool (see Kahneman, and Ariely for popular texts on the matter). One might even say we do not deploy the tool at all.

There are many problems with the standard model of expected value or expected utility that we have come across. Let's take a moment to sum them up here. We delved into the problem of precision and how that plays a role in the expected value calculations. It seems entirely unlikely we present the answer key to our values with that kind of precision.

Next, we discovered that the model is a decision tree to which there is no certain end. Where should one stop making these calculations? Thinking about where to prune this tree is going to be somewhat arbitrary. We will already be resorting to some rules of thumb. This appears to be contrary to the spirit of the EV model. We would be sneaking a lot of arbitrary numbers into the value part of the equation.

The best way to think about it is to imagine there are two kinds of risks. There is risk involved with having a negative outcome. It is a known risk. The probability is known, and so is the negative value. The gambling examples are good illustrations of these kinds of risks. Then there is the risk of not knowing all the variables that are involved. Uncertainty may involve some risk, but it also involves not knowing what variables may be in play. Many years of being involved with clinical research have given me a good understanding of these differences. When setting up a clinical trial that is considered the gold standard, you pick out what variables you would like to control. You do this on the basis that these variables could impact the result, and then you randomize among those variables. For example, you want both the test group, which is the group getting the drug, and the control group, which may be a placebo; you have similar proportions of gender, race, age, and so on. You are trying to minimize the influence these elements will have on the outcome of the drug experiment. The only influence on the outcomes of the experiment should be the test drug. We were hoping, for example, that if there are headaches in each group, that will wash out in the analysis. The placebo group will have, say, 1 percent of the patients having a headache. The drug group will have close to 1 percent having a headache. So, it did not make a difference whether or not you got the drug or the placebo. Similarly, improvements in your medical condition should only be attributable to which group you were in.

The randomization process is meant to reduce those headaches. You will normally randomize across age, various confounding medical conditions, and some other variables. Suppose the test drug group results in 5 percent of the patients getting a headache. The placebo group only had 1 percent of the patients getting a headache. You're led to believe, of course, that the headache must be due to the drug. However, when you look at who got placed in the placebo group and who got placed in the drug group, you find out that there are five times as many patients that have a history of headaches in the drug group. Now you don't know whether their extra headaches are due to the drug or their history of headaches. If you randomize the people coming in with variables that you think will be important and impactful, then you hope that there are equal numbers of those in each of the two groups. They sort of wash each other out. It might be that women have far more headaches than men. So, if one group has more women, there will be a problem. Randomly selecting people is meant to give essentially equivalent numbers in both groups.

You may have already guessed the problem that we face here. How do we know what variables to include? The expected value model wants to include all possible outcomes and their probabilities. That really does not seem applicable to a medical situation. In fact, it does not seem applicable to many real-world choice situations in life. The choice of variables to include is somewhat uncertain. There may be two probabilities at play here. One is the probability of known outcomes. The other is the uncertainty that we've collected all the probable outcomes. Gigerenzer has written extensively about this type of uncertainty. He has spent much of his career working on how to make good decisions when not all risks are known or calculable.

The Sum of Problems

There is the requirement of arithmetical values for each outcome. Generally, we don't have those values readily at hand. At best, we might be able to supply an order of one thing over another over another, and so on. This is known as an ordinal ranking. Psychologically we are capable of creating rank orderings. When we supply a rank order, it is more like taste preferences than currency.

Another significant issue for EVs is this idea of stopping rules. EV requires stopping rules on the decision tree. The final expected value is a sum of all the expected values calculated along the way. You need to sum each branch of the decision tree, and it needs to be followed to the very last twig, as in Figure 2 above. As the branches get longer, producing a decision becomes an arithmetical nightmare. Arithmetical equations are prone to error and, as a matter of practicality, should be avoided if we can. The gambling scenarios where these started have a natural stopping point.

Another challenge is one where we try to place numerical values on symptoms that oscillate between severe to less severe and back. The symptoms may affect functionality, and that would have to be considered. We would need to place numerical values on scales for each stopping point. For example, for my first round of nausea let us add a negative value of I-don't-know minus

22 on a scale of 100 and it lasted for seven hours. The next bout of nausea lasted for two hours, but that was judged as a minus seven, so I could take minus 22 * 7 and then minus 2 * 7, add those together, and continue to go down that branch. It is unclear whether I can forecast every branch to reach the same time points. There is also the challenge of judging how in the future I will feel about the nausea in that experience. That is, I don't know if I will become less sensitive, so to speak, to the nausea or more sensitive.

It will be prudent to search out other alternatives given these problems with the expected value model.

Alternative Decision-Making Models

Any alternative model still has to consider some things that the expected value model integrated into its paradigm. The tree diagram summed up all the intermediate outcomes, not just the final outcome. The ends don't necessarily justify the means. We will take this on when we review the case of Dax Cowart. It is a fantastic illustration of this. But first, let's look at an alternative model from the world of ethics.

Jeremy Bentham's Utilitarianism

So let us first look at decision-making models that have been previously published. One is that proposed by Jeremy Bentham back in 1780 and subsequently published in 1789. Bentham was an 18th-century British philosopher. He had broad interests, from reforming the British penal system to ethics. He was quite an important individual with respect to the British approach to jails and punishment, which he reformed from a punitive system to one of rehabilitation. His ventures into ethics made him one of the founders of Utilitarianism. His legacy includes his reconstructed skeleton with a wax head likeness dressed in his clothes. This is preserved in the University College of London. This all came about from instructions left in his will. What a legacy. What a school.

His approach is appealing because he wants a method for selecting outcomes that will generate the most happiness. It involves happiness as the value for the outcome, which is not dissimilar to our goals. It also involves likelihoods that resemble probabilities. Happiness, for Bentham, is the only value to consider. All other values can be reduced to it. His area was ethics, and he felt our choices should always be evaluated regarding how they affect the greater whole, not just ourselves. This led to the principle of utility, which is stated as "do that action which will promote the greatest happiness for the greatest number of people." Our goal is a bit more circumscribed. If we were going to use Bentham, we would be looking for that act that provides the greatest happiness for the patient. Let's call this version of Bentham "U2" (with my apologies to Bono).

Bentham argues that happiness is nothing more than pleasure. Pain and pleasure are the variables of interest. How do you measure pleasure? He suggests that there are four aspects to consider for a person by themselves. They are the intensity of the experience, its duration, certainty (or uncertainty), and propinquity or remoteness in time. The last two have more to do with whether the feelings are near at hand as opposed to a remote event. This is known as the hedonistic calculus.

Bentham doesn't really tell us how all this works together. He doesn't say for each individual how to integrate the variables mentioned. His interest was more in the amalgamation of each individual's pleasure and pain taken together with everyone else's. There he simply states that for the act, take each person's pleasure and add up that column, and for each person's pain add that column up. If the positive outweighs the negative, then you've got something good. Unfortunately, this isn't enough of a recipe for us. Still, it seems to be closer to how we really think. We will keep this alternative in mind, and perhaps we can fill in some of the blanks.

U2 incorporates items that we need to take into account, including the duration of the outcome, the intensity of the outcome, the probability of the outcome, and how close it is at hand. In some ways, it is really a more general version of the EV model without the restrictions of exact probabilities. Its generality is a double-edged sword. It leaves us room to supply details that avoid challenges from the EV model. Unfortunately, it also means that we need to supply the details ourselves.

The Fast and Frugal Method

The Fast and Frugal method is a third model of decision-making under uncertainty. Herbert Simon first developed the approach which he termed "bounded rationality." Gigerenzer was among those who came after Simon. Those following this line of reasoning objected to the incredibly complex requirements of the expected value model. It is certainly one of the complaints I have noted out for its use in this context. The authors and proponents of the Fast and Frugal camp focused on the practicality of decision-making. One must be careful, as these authors point out that the Fast and Frugal method is not universally the best method to apply (Gigerenzer and Gaissmaier). They wouldn't, for example, suggest that it is better for gambling scenarios than is the expected value method.

The Fast and Frugal method has allowed them to produce several approaches that use heuristics to generate better choices. A heuristic is an algorithm or procedural rule to follow. They have what I consider the laudable goal of making good choices and not being subservient to finding the best possible choice. The heuristics that they search for are quick methods that get you pretty darn good results. Unfortunately, the heuristics that they have only work under certain domains. Whether or not it can be applied to the medical context can be questioned.

One heuristic is the one-bounce rule. You keep going through your options so long as they improve. In the first downturn, stop searching, and take the last option that was an improvement. Of course, you need to know whether the option is or is not an improvement.

This methodology offers several other heuristics. We won't go into them here. What we do know is that any approach has to satisfy certain requirements. We have established that probabilities play a role in at least some circumstances. Personal preferences are essential. So, there must be a way for the decision model to incorporate those preferences. It also means that now we must be able to make comparisons to have preferences. One merely has to go back to the diner example to see that you have to be able to compare the menu items against one another to make a choice.

Fast and Frugal has more specificity than Bentham's model and more applicability than EV. I do not see how Fast and Frugal can handle values. Still, it might be useful in determining the relevance of the information for a patient. You will recall that a major issue with the informed consent paradigm is this inability to determine what information is relevant. One of the Fast and Frugal heuristics might look like the following: Suppose an HCP and a patient are getting started on therapeutic choices. The HCP could ask the patient to list the types of symptoms that bother them the most. Take the listing as a priority ranking, with the first one on the list being the most important. This relies on the hypothesis that one more easily recalls the most important priorities for themselves first. This can inform the HCP about the relevant symptoms to disclose as risks. You might want to add any high-probability risks even if they do not appear on the patient's list. This approach would need to be empirically tested.

The paradigm of choice needs to be supporting patient decision-making. To accomplish this, it will take a paradigm shift from throwing information over the transom to one involving sharing and support. Figuring out how to do this is quite a challenge. We have issues with comprehension of the information, determining the relevance of the information, relating it to our values, calculating probabilities, and diminished capacities throughout.

Summary of the Models

The jury is still out on these approaches. The expected value approach gives great answers to some problems, especially those associated with currency as the standard value. This seems problematic because the value we're seeking is not currency. We would be force-fitting scales to fill the role of currency. We would also be taking the calculations out in the branching of the decision tree to such an extent that we don't even know where we should stop. Although the expected value model is meant to be a normative model (that is, we *should* be using it, not that we do), it speaks against it if we can't use it.

One of its biggest flaws is that it doesn't really reflect how we think, even when we are thinking rationally. It also fails us on practical dimensions. This leaves us with another possibility. Either the model (EV) for rational thinking is too stringent, or we are not rational. Proponents of the theory as a guiding theory of rational thought would point out that this is how we should think and should be the standard by which we are judged. This is, of course, a possible approach. However, in my opinion, the circumstances in which this model is appropriate (and there are such circumstances) are a special case, and the model has more restrictions than a less rigorous model of rational thinking. I hope to illustrate and persuade you that there is a model for rational decision-making that is more general and yields sensible results given who we are and how we actually value experiences and outcomes. The expected utility model is a special case of the general model and works well—even better—in a certain decision-making domain. It is best to leave the EV for that domain.

The Utilitarian model has the advantage of being a bit more general on some of these items. I look at it as the general approach that is required to make good decisions, one that needs to apply to the domain of interest. In our case, it is the medical context we're interested in, and people's own personal values. If we were calculating five-year mortality rates, we would use something more akin to the expected value model. All the inputs are numeric. The values are objective and easily determined. They are life and death. We may have our personal views of how much life is worth, but five-year mortality rates don't speak to that. You are either dead or not. The value of each death is equal. Expected value would only work if we each had the same value in any possible outcome.

Did Jeremy Bentham's utilitarianism (U2) model offer a more general approach to decision-making under uncertainty? The short answer is yes. Yet it does not offer a lot of guidance on how to calculate anything. It is possible that we can supply enough of the inner workings to make it go of this approach. We don't want to go overboard, as in the EV model, but it does seem to be a lightweight version of it. There is yet another decision model we can leverage that would be quick and offer a little more meat on the bones of Jeremy Bentham's version of utilitarianism adapted for our purpose.

Paradigms Revisited

Let us fill out the paradigms. At this point, the informed consent paradigm has the features of one-way communication from physician to patient. The information itself is highly technical. It involves communicating probabilities of various outcomes. The communication struggles about which of the myriad outcomes need to be communicated. Because the information is technical and couched in scientific terminology, much work was done (Richards) on patients' comprehension of the information given and the work continues (Glaser). It is especially difficult to inform patients about risks (Wegwarth).

This is an extremely important point because paradigms in their worldviews dictate what is important to do. Certainly, patient comprehension is necessary under any of the paradigms that may be suggested; however, with informed consent, it is the only thing that requires the health care provider to do some extra work. There is little focus on values clarification. This is seen to be in the province of the patient, not the health care provider. Manson and O'Neill would describe this as the container approach to communication (viii). As such, it has been part and parcel of the IC paradigm. I often think about it as the physician puts the information in the tube and throws it over a wall. The patient picks it up and decides. The patient then inserts their choice in the tube and throws it back to the health care provider.

There are also social aspects to the paradigm. The physician controls the information. She or he could present it in ways that would lead the patient to a particular choice. Information is power. How the choices are described and communicated all play a role. Informed consent leaves the power to the health care provider. When we make patient information an essential element of the interaction, the power is also shared. Inspecting the informed consent paradigm, the only question typically asked is "do you have any questions?" followed by a response as to which of the various selections they would like to pursue.

The shared decision-making paradigm has shown itself to be more inclusive in several ways. Under this paradigm, the patient regains some of the power. It also bestows upon the patient some responsibilities. They need to help the physician sort out what is important to disseminate.

What is the information that the patient is sharing? It is their values. It is no wonder that the SDM paradigm explores value clarification for the patient. Several models and exercises for value clarification have been put in place since shared decision-making has come to the forefront.

This brings us to the question of how we generate our preferences or values. I'm not going to go into the philosophical depths of this discussion. For the purposes of this book, I will just go with the hypothesis that we each have some predisposition to prefer certain things over others. These preferences are very flexible over time and across individuals. I like chocolate, you like vanilla. As they say, "There is no accounting for taste." This approach will allow us to focus on information and its relationship to our experiences. Who better to tell our story than Goldilocks?

Goldilocks and Packaging

You might find it strange to rely on a fairy tale, but it illustrates well how information needs to be packaged to resonate with a patient. The Goldilocks fable gives us some extra insight into why we might want to restrict the right of autonomy to adults as well. The story of Goldilocks is a well-known fairytale. To remind those who haven't heard it in a while, the story begins in the home of the three bears. They are Papa Bear, Mama Bear, and Baby Bear. They have just made some porridge, but it is too hot to eat. The bears leave to take a walk to let it all cool off. Shortly after their departure, Goldilocks arrives a bit hungry and tired. She sizes up the situation as she is confronted with choices. There are three chairs, three bowls of porridge, and three beds. As it turns out, she is both curious and a poor decision-maker. Let us focus on two of the situations confronting her: three bowls of mush. She must choose one that she will be able to tolerate. She has information, but it is visual information that yields little clue as to taste or temperature. Eating it will provide the experiential information needed for taste and temperature. They are the variables that need to be accounted for, and she receives no information about any of them by simply looking.

She looks at the bowls of porridge and chooses the Papa Bear bowl. She takes a taste, and it is too hot. Then she selects the Mama Bear bowl, tastes that porridge, and it is too cold. She finally settles in on the Baby Bear's bowl, and the porridge is just right.

When Goldilocks goes upstairs, she looks at the beds and must choose which one is the most comfortable. In this case, it requires that the information be tactile. Her data now is still visual. Again, she sorts through the information through trial and error. Mostly in error, as she always guesses wrong on the first two attempts. It is only through experience that Goldilocks can process the information appropriately.

She will need to experience the choices to get to the right answer. In each case, she simply tries them out. She will taste the bowls of porridge or sit in the beds.

We can surmise that Goldilocks is extremely poor at guessing. Always two wrong guesses before arriving at the right choice. A few comments are in order here. The decision problem for Goldilocks is based on her sensory preferences. A certain range of temperatures for porridge and a certain sense of firmness of the mattress. This cannot be emphasized enough that she will compare experiences to make her best decision. In her circumstances, the actual "testing" is not particularly harmful. Will the porridge she selected potentially burn her mouth, which would obviously be disastrous? Experiencing the alternatives, especially in such close succession, is particularly advantageous. This, we must point out, is not the typical consent situation in choosing medical interventions. "We will just try the surgery first and see how that feels." That does not sound like a particularly good plan. I would rather get the information in language without having to go through the experience if possible.

In our settings, we are reluctant to utilize the Goldilocks experimental method. The choices can have side effects that are too severe to risk. Although, again, this may not apply to all cases. Many decisions can be reversed later with less than disastrous consequences. In these cases, the question is which therapy to choose. For Goldilocks, facing the porridge bowls and looking at them (the same is true of the beds) does not offer any information relevant to her preferences. It would make a difference if she were picking out art. Then the visual information will be all telling. Alas, this is not the case here.

If we want to make it similar, we must encourage verbalizing the differences in the temperature in the bowls of porridge (or verbalizing the firmness of the beds.) Sounds easy till you try. Looking at the porridge, it turns out that its perceived warmth is the key. How do you tell Goldilocks about the heat of the porridge so she can relate it to her preferences? Similarly, as a health care provider, how would you inform a patient about the different interventions if they have not been through any of them in the past? Let's start with Goldilocks.

One approach is to relay the information in terms of temperature. We could say the Papa bowl is 180°F and the Mama bowl is 65°F. The baby bowl is 120°F. What does this mean for Goldilocks? This sort of information is a lot like the information that is given in the informed consent context in that it is both objective and very quantitative.

Now the ball is in Goldilocks' court. Exactly how would she process this information? She must be able to make a connection between the information and what she has experienced knowing about those temperatures. If she has not had the experience of relating Fahrenheit readings with heat sensation in her mouth, then it would not be relevant to inform her of the temperature in this way.

We can tell how hard this is on the HCP too. Goldilocks will have to relate the temperature information in degrees Fahrenheit (or centigrade if she was born outside of the US) to a memory of heat that has already been correlated with the temperature. In other words, if someone has already had the oral sensation and was told at the same time the degrees Fahrenheit, they would be able to make a correlation. Personally, even when I have burned the roof of my mouth with pizza, I couldn't tell you how hot it was in terms of degrees Fahrenheit. No one ever told me. Now, as adults, we might remember that our body temperature is at 98.6°F, and water boils at 212°F. The latter sounds too hot, but I know 98.6° will be somewhat tepid. That is quite a gap. I confess that I have no idea what temperature in between would feel best to me.

In terms of experience and background knowledge, I have an advantage over Goldilocks. She may not have knowledge of core body temperature or the temperature of boiling water or hot coffee or the pizza cheese burning the roof of her mouth. And lo and behold, it is hard to see how she would be able to make sense of the information without making the connection between the data and the experience, so she will be able to assign to it if she doesn't have this prior experience.

The confrontation with the beds makes me feel somewhat like how Goldilocks would feel about hearing the temperature readings. I have no knowledge of firmness information except for soft and hard, neither of which appeals to me. This information about the firmness (hard or soft) is not so objective. As it turns out, mattress manufacturers do have measures of firmness. These are scales. However, I do not know the scales in terms of experience. It might be a genuinely nice one to ten type of scale. However, I don't know if these scales are linear. That is, I don't know if the differences between a five and a seven are the same as the difference between a seven and nine. I can't relate the scale to my preferences until I sit or lie in bed and am told the firmness number. Experience with relevant information makes us wiser in our choices.

Challenges to Informing Well

The Goldilocks dilemma above is only one of many challenges of informing patients well. Just as patient preferences may be unique, so is their ability to meaningfully relate the information to their experience. If the patient has never had the experience of one of the outcomes of importance, it is hard to see how well they can process that information.

There are other issues with providing appropriate information to patients. As we saw in the diner experience, words that have no meaning, such as the item's proper name, provide no relevance for the consumer. Likewise, technical polysyllabic words were never meant for the lay public.

The health care provider faces some challenges in giving the information to the patient. The courts were correct when they feared information overload getting in the way of proper communication. Behavioral economics has a rather long list of ways that we can mess up the use of information in making choices under uncertainty.

Several biases typically occur when we process information rapidly. There are good reasons for us to process information rapidly most of the time. We would be worse off if we did EV calculations every time we had to choose during the day. My guess is we would likely starve to death or, at the very least, be tossed out of the diner.

Kahneman and others have termed the two modes of thinking as system one and system two (17). These systems incorporate more than conceptual processing. They include physiological responses, behaviors, and perceptions. I would like to restrict this to our intake of information. Let's call them "Think One" and "Think Two" (my apologies to Doctor Seuss). Think One processes information rapidly and looks for a heuristic to make decisions—no need to calculate here. Think Two is the opposite and is typified by the calculations and the expected value model. It is a lot like calculating through chess or balancing a checkbook.

Fast and Frugal is more of a Think One type of process. It doesn't look to be instantaneous as in Gladwell's Blink, but it is meant to be simple, quick, and yield pretty good choices. It works by triggering associative machinery. It restricts itself to the right cues. If somebody says the word "banana" to me, I also think of the term yellow. If somebody mentions a hero of mine, I will place great characteristics around that individual.

These diverse ways of approaching decisions play a role in the types of information required. We shall see later that the ethics of the situation demands that we be competent at making decisions. It is, therefore, necessary to understand which model we're using to test if we're any good at it. The goal of the decision-making model will be that it leads to good decisions. Of course, we understand this, which is a basic assumption when we employ it. The fact there are different decision-making models available is overlooked much of the time. We just jump right in and figure our way through things without stepping back. As an illustration of a personal nature, I typically use my salary and projected raises when I project my future earnings. I then use math to figure out how much I will earn. I won't make an intuitive guess.

On the other hand, when I am selecting whether to hit a forehand or a backhand in tennis, I do not start calculating trajectories and angles. My experience and quick decision-making take hold. Unfortunately, I am only average at the latter.

As far as the decision-making models go, they have some similar challenges and some that are uniquely their own. In fact, there is much overlap in the challenges between them. There are biases in how we absorb information that make the models less fruitful. A lot of these have been detailed by several authors and researchers in behavioral economics. A look at the notes in Kahneman is richly populated with resources. I won't tread over the same ground except to highlight a few examples for you.

Examples of Biases

There are problems with giving too much information. It makes it difficult to discriminate between what is important and what is not. Given that part of this is to trigger associative machinery, perhaps too much stimulation leads to nothing coming to the forefront. The idea here is that there are too many associations to be triggered, so none get triggered. Nothing will stand out. This is another reason the patients apply value information before having all the alternatives. It is simply too much to sort all the possibilities like in our decision tree. Think Two is out of the question. Think One requires that only a few alternatives are considered. The trick is picking out which ones.

It is possible to rely on what most patients have reported as being important to them. I see this as a fallback position when the patient cannot express a preference order after some value clarification. This will make it a little dicey in protecting the patient's autonomy, as it isn't necessarily the case that you prefer things as others do. It will be critical to discuss the journey along the way. In fact, the journey itself is a series of intermediate outcomes. If you were following an EV analysis, you would calculate each of those in your final totals.

Expressing probabilities is another issue, as it seems we are all lacking proficiency in anything involving mathematics. We have already taken issue with the idea of precise probabilities even being necessary, since our valuation of the outcomes is not nearly that precise. However, we do know some things about the idea of likelihood. It does appear that when the difference in probabilities is rather large, we can handle the information. Expressing those probabilities in a meaningful way by the health care practitioner is extremely important. Gerd Gigerenzer has been widely published on the topic of risk communication under uncertainty (Risk Savvy).

One of the issues in communicating risks is that there are two types of risks commonly used in the medical literature. One is the absolute risk of an event happening. The other is a relative risk, which is the risk compared to another known risk. An example would be a therapy that reduces risk by 50 percent. This sounds great (it is) and impactful, which it might not be. Suppose the usual death rate is two in one million people. The therapy reduces this death rate to 1 in 1 million people. When the rates are so minuscule, the reduction of 50 percent is no longer as impactful. To be frank, most people would likely ignore this as progress, as it seems like a rounding error in magnitude. Alternatively, if the current death rate was 6000 out of one million, then the reduction by 50 percent saves 3000 people. It makes a difference. This has been pointed out by Gigerenzer (Gigerenzer, Risk pp. 16-18; 155; 179-188). It is the difference between an absolute risk and a relative risk. We do better with absolute risks.

How should we do it? Let's start with how we shouldn't do it. We shouldn't be using decimals as a way of transmitting risk information or probabilities. We can't typically process this numerical data unless we are using Think Two thinking. Since Think Two thinking typically involves values that are also decimal-like (as in our expected value model), its precision can get in the way. However, we can think in terms of percentages or using visual imagery.

One approach is to use a seating chart of a large stadium and reserve the right proportion of seats that reflect the likelihood of the outcome rather than a decimal number. I imagine myself sitting in a stadium with 1000 other people. I am told that one of us will suffer a heart attack. Compare this to sitting in a room with five people, and I am told one of us will have a heart attack. I'd rather have a ticket at the stadium. Following this approach, we get a better sense of how important the risk is to us in terms of its likelihood. In some ways, combining it with the value helps me keep the feelings front and center. I will have to combine the sense of risk with the value of that risk. The outcome of integrating the two must give me a rank order. In other words, we seek results that say one option is better. That's it. We are not seeking that option A is, say, 20 percent better than option B.

The bias we possess and the errors we typically perform are numerous. In *Thinking Fast and Slow*, Kahneman has different sections or chapters devoted to less-than-successful attempts to deal with information. They range from lazy executive function through availability to an inability to deal with different statistical pieces of information.

The remaining issues with the information have more to do with the reception of the patient in greater detail, as well as the miscalculations we might make as a result. They are not necessarily mistakes of information regarding what is relevant or digestible. These are more unwanted biases generated by how the information is conveyed, including the setting. After all, we want to make this as good as practically possible.

This work focuses on the two paradigms of informed consent and shared decision-making. We will not be reviewing the work of behavioral economists for every pitfall. I do believe, though, that it is instructive to look at a couple of categories of error-making that play a role in either paradigm.

The pandemic serves as a wonderful example of our lack of health literacy. It was problematic determining how to express to the public the danger of the virus. It is complicated because it requires an idea of how respiratory viruses spread and an understanding of probabilistic notions. We have seen how hard it is to deal with probabilities, and we always want to default to cause and effect.

The information coming out of the US Government was all over the place. Instead of explaining to people that the situation had too many unknowns to give directions to what we should exactly do, it offered conflicting information. There were too many unknowns initially other than that the virus seemed to be very deadly and easily transmitted. In my opinion, a sobering approach would have been more simplistic. We should have said it is apparently a severe virus that causes ICU-type interventions and may lead to many deaths. We want to ensure we don't overwhelm our health care system to the extent that we can't treat people who need treatment. Whether it's from the virus or heart attacks, or other problems. The spread of the disease and the seriousness of the complications all indicate that we must do something in the near term to stop the spread. Wearing masks will help, and it is our only device currently. The better the mask, the more protection.

At this point, health education might step in with more details. Maybe a visual explanation of particles coming out of someone's mouth, looking like a dense cloud and slowly dissipating to fewer and fewer molecules. The idea would be that you would like to minimize the number of molecules getting into your mouth. Series of visuals could be devised to display that idea, showing that you're safe if you're nowhere near the particles. The closer you come, then the more you need to present a barrier to the particles. If both parties wear masks, fewer particles can get out to be available to come into your mouth. In this way, you have articulated a lot of probabilistic numbers and how many feet and so on. It is like the problem we have explaining difficult probabilistic concepts in the consent arena. What you don't want are mixed messages with either dire predictions of a causal nature or overly optimistic ones. We got both, and though everyone wanted firm answers, the fact is that at the beginning, we were under maximum uncertainty. If you are portraying certainty, you'd better be right. The fact that the populace suffers from health illiteracy contributes to the problem. "Does the virus cause death?" "Will the vaccine prevent death and hospitalization?" What is missing from these questions is what people are asking: "Will the vaccine prevent my death or my hospitalization?" And they want a yes or no answer. Not one couched in probabilities.

Errors in Making Choices

Over the past 50 years, behavioral economics has amply demonstrated that we do not manage information extremely well. We are prone to making errors or being influenced by how the information is delivered. I like to think some of it's due to the packaging and some of it's due to the environment. Here is a short list of things we do wrong when processing information and how it impacts the choice between paradigms.

We lack the stamina to think things through. We will opt out of an effortful problem to substitute something simpler. If we are going to help the patient make a good decision, we cannot make the choice an endurance test. Whether they are health care providers or patients, decision-makers will not tolerate complex, cumbersome decision-making. The bounded rationality models, Fast and Frugal, would be the preferred norm under these circumstances.

It takes effort to make decisions. The effort is both physical and mental. Patient capacity for this is diminished potentially by their physical condition. It is also easy to be distracted from the task at hand. There are a few things, as health care providers, we can do to mitigate this fact.

We need to provide an atmosphere that is conducive to thinking about just the problem. It takes effort not to be distracted. Interruptions are not invited. The physical environment should be as comfortable as possible.

Information can prime us to trigger an umbrella of concepts. Pictures of people over a collection dish for coffee will result in more donations (Bateson pp. 412-414). It is as if a real person is watching us. Money priming also results in and motivates more independence and selfishness on the part of the participant. This may be one place where that is an excellent idea. Gestures have similar consequences. If we smile at somebody, it will lift their mood. It is not clear to me, at least, how we should behave with this understanding. What physical environment will hopefully help a patient make a better decision? Should you smile? Should you frown?

Familiarity with a word or phrase makes it appear to be true. We have recently seen in our politics quite a bit of repetition resulting in belief. The more repetition, the stronger the belief. Perhaps one of the approaches should be to repeat through the patient's alternatives and the likelihood of their outcomes.

Some of our other foibles include jumping to conclusions, believing in causality, and confirmation bias. To deal with these, the HCP needs to be an active listener to determine if the patient is engaging in any of these activities.

The fact that we are dealing with likelihood means that we are not dealing with a causal nexus unless the likelihoods are approaching 100 percent. This may go hand in hand with jumping to conclusions rather than tapping on the brakes a bit. One can also test for confirmation bias by having the patient articulate how they came to a decision. A patient who has just heard the word "cancer" may immediately jump to the conclusion that they are going to die, and they will stop listening to a lot of the other data being presented because it doesn't fit their conclusions.

The order of presentation makes a difference. If something is presented first, it is deemed to be more important. The framing of the information is also relevant. We treat potential losses as being more important than potential gain. Studies have shown that whether it be the physician or the patient, we feel differently about losses and gains. This harkens back a bit to Bernoulli. It is not clear to me how to deal with this feature of our human intellect. It is like talking about a cash discount versus a credit surcharge. In our case, it may be something like comparing the two sentences "you are going to live for two more years" versus "you're going to die in two more years." Perhaps stating it both ways may help, but cognitive studies need to be employed to help figure this out.

One feature of the system here between the two types of thinking is most critical. This means you will have to use Think One no matter what. Think One translates values across dimensions. This is how we compare our seemingly dissimilar categories of values to one another. Behavioral experiments have compared height to intelligence (Kahneman 101 of 570). The challenge would be comparing, say, IQ to height. Suppose a basketball player is seven feet tall, and you want to compare that to the IQ of people in your class. You know intuitively that a seven-foot-tall person is quite unusual. If you know that IQ ranges from, say, 70 to 160, then how smart are those who are similar to the seven-foot-tall person? You are probably going to guess above 140. We must make these sorts of decisions all the time when we're rank-ordering preferences. We might be comparing the length of life versus the quality of life over a shorter period. We might be comparing the pleasure we get from reading a book over the pleasure we get from going to a restaurant and eating. Somehow, we do this all the time. The process is intuitive and falls under Think One.

So far, the journey has led us to favor a Fast and Frugal methodology or, more generally, a bounded rationality approach. Now, let us summarize where we stand with the paradigms and the decision models by comparing them in Table 1 below.

Table 1 Comparison of Paradigms for the Patient HCP Interaction

Informed Consent	Shared Decision Making
Information flows one way HCP to patient	Information flows two ways
Information is factual and arithmetic	Information is factual, and values (less precise if at all)
Failed because of lacking patient input	Requires patient input
EV friendly	Bounded Rationality friendly, fast, and frugal, Bentham like
Can be done quickly	Burdensome on staff approach
Poor patient compliance	Improved patient compliance
Paternalistic	Power Sharing – More friendly to patient autonomy

To this point, the assumption has been that shared decision-making better supports autonomy. There is an important domain yet to be investigated, which is really the foundation of what has gone above. We must deal with the ethics of the situation because that gives rise to the patient's autonomy. Somehow, in some way, we need to come to a decision about the meaning of autonomy in this context. I cannot think of a better way to deal with two vivid and important cases that involve patient autonomy versus paternalism. We'll start with the oldest and undoubtedly the most famous case of all.

Chapter 4

We Need to Listen

Schloendorff

At the time, she was Mary Gamble, a teacher of physical training voice culture, reduction, and development. Mary was born in Oregon in the 1850s, though records were scarce as Oregon was a territory at the time. She lived in San Francisco for most of her life. Yet, nothing would have predicted the next sequence of events in her life. There are no clear census records concerning where she lived in San Francisco or with whom she lived. Mr. Gamble does not appear to be in the picture in 1906. Mary was about 52 years old at the time. She had two sons, Evan and Thaddeus (or Theodore). Evan was living in Manhattan. He was an actor in 1910 and eventually married Hortense P— a descendant and member of the Daughters of the American Revolution. Theodore was the manager of a firm and was selling hair tonic. Mary's health was fine.

This all changed on April 18th, 1906. It was pretty early in the morning (5:13 a.m.). Her world was about to fall apart. It felt like awakening on a bed of Jell-O. Then came the loud crashes. Shock and panic set in. The thunderous roar of buildings collapsing on themselves was bad enough, but the fires that ensued were worse by measure. Close to a half million inhabitants were in the city. A truly beautiful city with a hotel costing 3 million dollars back in the early 1900s, worth about 70 million dollars today. What most don't know is that even though the entire city rests on a rock, a layer of sand acts as a buffer against the shock. To say that panic ensued would be an understatement. Springs in San Francisco were temperate. Well, the weather is constant all year round, usually in the 50s. But on April 18th at

5:13 a.m., the air above ground didn't signify any changes. It was beneath the ground that massive fronts would collide.

How long would such an event take? Well, I suppose a lot would depend upon what you count as the event. The quake itself—the initial tremors— nothing but a few seconds for the first shock. The shock of being awakened from sleep and getting one's bearings in what must have seemed like awakening from a dream state into a nightmare. Walls falling, ceilings and floors caving in, and loud explosions from the city outside.

The subsequent aftershocks were even more frightful. The world seemed to cave in on itself as beds were swallowed up by the floor, which was being swallowed by the ground beneath like some Russian doll set. The tremors continued with the worst one at 8 a.m. Having already experienced their fortification tumbling, this tremor, though not the most forceful at first, found its weakened structures and frightened populace ripe for devastation.

Gravity worked its cruel force upon the city, bringing structures down on and around its inhabitants. But the worst was yet to come. As if to provide a malevolent symmetry to the falling buildings, flames rose into the air everywhere in the tinder-laden city. Embers from evening fires had now engaged with the early morning falling wood to unite in a city-wide conflagration. Desperate measures were employed to slow the progress of the fire. People created a fire line by dynamiting the buildings in the blaze's path. Water was scarce—an odd thing for a town on a bay, but the quake had destroyed the water pipes beneath the ground. The only places that had water were the areas right along the bay itself where water could be pumped from the bay. All was done to quench the thirst of the fire.

This was the environment that people were faced with. The inhabitants created a mass exodus from the affected areas. The Presidio and Golden Gate Park areas were the people's destinations.

A reminder of a city catastrophe would include elements of Hurricanes Katrina and Sandy in terms of devastation and seeking safe ground. However, the events of 9/11 also ring familiar to elements of being caught up by the fire and the search for loved ones. In San Francisco, soldiers were called out to restore order and some measure of safety during the quake. They prevented people from rushing back into the crumbling buildings to save valuables and dear possessions. "At Larking and Sutter streets two men and a woman broke from the police and rushed into a burning apartment house, never to reappear" (Morris, p. 915 of 5025).

Most reminiscent of 9/11 was the report of Max Fast: "When the fire caught the Windsor Hotel at Fifth and Market Streets, there were three men on the roof, and it was impossible to get them down. Rather than see the crazed men fall in with the roof and be roasted alive, the military officer directed his men to shoot them, which they did in the presence of 5000 people" (Morris, p. 822 of 5025). The view we have of those actions is interesting. The officer's action has a benevolent favor —a mercy killing.

Similarly, for those who have seen the film *Last of the Mohicans*, there is a rather gruesome scene where the British officer is being burned at the stake. Shooting him seems like the best thing to do, and this action does not diminish our opinion of Hawkeye. It might even be enhanced. It is important to remember these behaviors and your own reaction to them when we analyze the behavior of the physicians in the Schloendorff v. Society of New York Hospital case. The intent to help and be benevolent is strong. It can be misguided when the good we try to implement is a projection of our notion of what "good," is rather than the person we are trying to help.

The situation near the ferries was equally panic-stricken. The flames prevented access to the pier for many. In their state of anxiety, some had to be held back from rushing into the fire to escape from them.

Though the park was able to provide refuge from falling objects and the ravaging flames, it could not provide for the other necessities of life. People slept on bare ground with little protection from the elements. In essence, there was no shelter, food, or water. The situation removed one other element from normal life: social standing was obliterated.

Back in the formerly inhabited city, death was everywhere. It was impossible not to be a witness to it.

One eyewitness reported, "at Seventh and Howard streets, a great lodging house took fire after the first shock before the guests had escaped. There were few exits, and nearly all the lodgers perished. Ms. JJ Munson, one of the individuals in the building, leaped with her child in her arms from the second floor to the pavement below and escaped unhurt. She says she was the only one who escaped" (Morris 1235 of 5025).

Over 3000 people died, and property losses would be equivalent to 6 billion dollars in 2011. The disaster clearly drove some insane, and had the diagnosis of post-traumatic stress disorder existed, it could no doubt have been applied to many of the survivors. Added to the misery was the fact that many had been separated from the rest of their families. There was no way to tell if a relative was merely separated from a loved one, had died in the quake, or was consumed by flames.

Mary Gamble was a resident of the city of San Francisco at the time of the earthquake. It is somewhat difficult to get a thoroughly confirmed picture of Mary before the quake. According to her testimony in court, she was "a teacher of physical training, voice culture, of reduction and development. Her physical condition in the fall of 1906 was, I might say, perfect" (Schloendorff para.49). By all accounts, she was born in the Oregon territory in the 1850s. She stated during the trial that her maiden name was Berry. Census records for Oregon in that period are pretty sketchy, but there is a record of Mary A Berry being born in 1854 or so. Future census records appear to shift, her birthdate, and place of origin. Now it is only important to mention that she was around 52 to 54 years old at the time of these events.

The *Western Journal of Education* lists a Mary E. Gamble in its 1903 register living in Almeda. In any case, she, by all accounts, was living comfortably. Her son Evan was living in New York at the time of the earthquake. There is never a mention of her husband. He is not listed as a fatality in the earthquake or a survivor. Mary is listed as a survivor. Other US and New York census data does not provide any more insight into Mr. Gamble. For whatever reason, he is no longer in the picture. Nor are Mary's parents the Berrys.

It is clear there is not enough information to establish whether Mary had post-traumatic stress disorder (PTSD). Nor is there enough information to establish her veracity because of inconsistent testimony on her part. We know that she was living in San Francisco during the time of the earthquake, and she admitted that this upset her nerves and caused her anxiety. This is important in painting a picture of Mary from two differing views. One is that of a frightened but perfectly cogent patient who complied with doctors' advice and clearly communicated her wishes, which were subsequently ignored. Her rights were trampled upon, and to add injury to insult, the intervention led to some awful consequences which were not handled professionally.

The other somewhat opposing picture is that she was nervous and inconsistent. Perhaps she even intentionally deceived others about who she was and had a long history of such deceptions, so that she gave contradictory information to the health care team and did not have a fully competent mind. Her behavior post-operatively was against all medical instruction, and her anxiety was so great that she was probably not of sound mind.

I do not mean to suggest that either is the actual truth. There is not enough information to make that determination with certainty. The truth is much closer to Mary's view, but I want to make the extremes plausible for illustration purposes rather than historical accuracy.

Mary's appearance in court made the papers of May 4th, 1911. It ran in the *New York Times* and the *Daily World*. Her picture illustrates a very composed and dignified lady. You would note her fashionable attire and her hands covered by gloves. She also, by this time, had remarried in New York. She relates her version of events and her state of mind during her testimony.

She stated she was in good physical health until April 1906. It was the great earthquake in San Francisco. "Well, I was greatly frightened and nervous, of course" (para. 49). It led to her departure to join her son in Manhattan. She stayed with him for a month until she took a room about a block away on West 117th street. She had pains in her stomach and was taking Stewart's dyspeptic tablets and Bromo Seltzer. She saw a doctor, Dr. Garlock, who advised her that she would later be admitted to the hospital.

Quite apart from the ethical components of these decisions is the state of medical science and practice at that time. Stuart's dyspeptic tablets were eventually taken off the market in 1933 for having absolutely no symptomatic or curative effect. At one point, they claimed to replace the digestive substances in the stomach, such as acid and pepsin. In all actuality, they were composed of some different carbonates and ginger. Bromo Seltzer at the time included a substance called Bromide (hence the name), a class of tranquilizers that may have contributed to their effect. Early forms also contained acetanilide, an early analgesic and fever-controlling substance. It had some severe toxicities associated with it, but when metabolized also produced the active substance in acetaminophen (Tylenol). Bromo Seltzer contains different ingredients today.

Nevertheless, we must remind ourselves that the FDA was not in existence at this time and that drugs were unregulated except for commerce itself. The medical profession had little in the way of tools to combat issues. Indeed, even Mary's procedure was experimental in those days.

Mary went to the hospital to receive treatment for the stomach ailment. Her son went with her. She had not lost her strength as of then. She arrived on Jan 10th, 1907. Her son spoke to a man at the desk who sent for a doctor. The good Dr. Bartlett was brought in to meet Evan. He told the doctor that he wanted to enter his mother as a patient because of stomach trouble. Evan asked how much it would cost, and the answer was seven dollars for the week (another anachronism, for sure). The good Dr. Garlock has already made arrangements for Mary's admission. Mary was assigned to Ward 1.

The hospital was interesting on its merit. It was The Society of New York Hospital. It is the second oldest hospital in the United States (Pennsylvania Hospital being the oldest). In 1769 Dr. Bard established that there was a need for a hospital for the poor.

Dr. Bartlett set about treating Mary for her stomach problems. He washed her stomach out every day. This was done using a nasogastric tube. He placed her on a regimen of raw egg and milk. This went on for three weeks. He had proclaimed her cured after two weeks but offered her the opportunity to stay for another week, as she had lost a lot of strength by this point in time.

She met Doctors Stimson and Cottle during her first week in the hospital. You see, Dr. Bartlett had discovered a lump upon examination of Mary and wanted a second opinion. Mary stated that she had had that lump for about five years. It seemed to come and then go away. According to Mary's account, Stimson said he could not find it upon exam. She thought and testified that

Bartlett said he had found it there the day before and that perhaps it was a tumor or a phantom tumor. Mary seemed to remember this in detail. She heard Stimson say that maybe it was a "floating kidney" (para. 58). She also apparently overheard Dr. Stimson tell the other doctors that she might have a "phantom tumor" (para. 58). Bartlett then attempted to find it upon exam, and it wasn't there again. This is when the two parties truly begin to diverge on what happened. According to Mary, "Dr. Stimson said that he could not find it, that I was too nervous, too rigid, or too tense. That he would have to have an ether examination to locate it" (para. 59).

Mary didn't understand what was meant by another examination, so the next time she saw Dr. Bartlett, she enquired about its meaning. He said "it meant to give the patient a little ether to quiet the nerves and relax the body. That it didn't amount to anything; and I told him 'I don't want any operation, Doctor'" (para. 60).

This did not end the discussion concerning ether and its suitability for Mary. She worried about her ability to take the anesthetic. She confirmed for Bartlett that she had taken chloroform and laughing gas in the past without any issues arising. She then relayed that Bartlett stated that since she tolerated these gases, ether was less dangerous and that "he advised me to—while I was in the hospital and was accessible to the surgeon, to simply find out what the operation—what the lump was; it would be a satisfaction to know what it was. Then, if anything required operation, I could return at any time if I wished to… I spoke to Dr. Bartlett several times in relation to my forbidding an operation. He said he did not advise any operation. He only advised an examination to determine the cause of that—he said it would be a satisfaction to know what the lump was about the middle of last week I was there" (para. 62).

What transpired next is one of three believable scenarios. A miscommunication between Bartlett and Mary. He was under the assumption that she had agreed to an ether exam, but the date was not agreed upon in advance. Bartlett had told her she could go at any time, but there is no testimony that she told Bartlett she was leaving the following day. Nor had she refused the exam. It is quite possible that Bartlett thought she had agreed to the exam and set it up for the following day. That the exam was set for the next morning is evident in that Mary was transferred to another ward that night, and the nurse told her that she would have an ether exam the following day. Mary stated that she had told the nurses that she was being discharged the next day. According to Mary, the nurses acknowledged that she was going for an ether examination the next day and that she showed Mary a slip of paper that read "Mrs. Gamble, ether examination." After being shown this piece of paper, Mary felt relief and submitted to the preparation.

So here we have a rather clear example of rather unclear communication. At least if we abide by the testimony as being a true rendering of the events. Mary was told she would have an ether exam. It seems that Mary considered that this exam would not involve any surgery. This is made abundantly clear when she tells the nurses that she will be discharged the following day. It is also clear that the physicians thought otherwise. And there was no testimony that anyone disputed her understanding. This is instructive in terms of checking what patients understand. Assumptions are dangerous in the communication.

"My body was swathed in antiseptic cloths; I was tied up like a mummy and placed back on the bed. I went to sleep. In the morning, the bandages had become displaced, and they were replaced. Then I was, about seven o'clock, given a cup of coffee" (para. 69).

She was then taken on an elevator on a pushcart. Accompanying her was one man; according to her testimony, what happens next is terrifying.

"I asked him what he was going to do, and he said he was going to give me gas. I says, 'What for?' He says, 'We always give gas preparatory to giving ether because ether often nauseates the patient and frightens them, so we give gas first.' And I says, 'What are they going to do me? Are they going to operate on me?' And he says, 'I don't know, I am simply detailed to give gas, that is all; I don't know.' 'But,' I says, 'I want to see somebody—show me somebody, I want to tell them I am not to be operated on.' And he says, 'Did you come for operation?' I said, 'No.' Then he says: 'You will not be operated on if you did not come in for an operation.' 'No,' I said, 'I came in for an ether examination.' He says, 'Then you will only receive an ether examination.' But I was frightened and tried to get up; I tried to get off the litter and get away.

And he pushed me—I could only raise my hand; all this time I was frightened and nervous. He had some apparatus there with a rubber tube and mouthpiece, and he took his hand and pushed against my forehead and pushed me back, and put the mouthpiece to my mouth and said, 'Take a deep breath.' 'I was frightened at the gas and tried to get up, took a deep breath, I guess, and did not know any more. I do not know who operated on me except by hearsay'" (para. 70-72).

What a surreal scene described by Mary. A few protestations were made to various people about her wishes. There was no evidence given to her of there being a course other than the one she approved—if we can even say she approved. Though not borne out in the testimony per se, Mary was certainly wise to be skeptical of her caretakers. Here she had thought she was going home the following day, and suddenly, she was being whisked away for a prep that no one had bothered to tell her about. Instead of the health care team telling Mary what was happening, she had to keep asking them. This certainly set up a context that could easily be interpreted as deceitful and misleading. At least this is one coherent picture based on Mary's testimony alone. Throughout the testimony given by Mary, the fact that the surgeon only saw her once leaves open the option, but very little was communicated from one doctor to another.

Another coherent picture is that of a mismanaged situation. No malice intended, but a lot of incompetency is transpiring. Dr. Bartlett is not clear to Mary that he wants her to stay for the next day for the "ether examination," or he is not clear in his orders to the staff that there is not going to be an ether exam the following day. Or, perhaps, there is a miscommunication between Dr. Stimson and Dr. Bartlett about the next steps. It could very possibly be that Bartlett had let Stimson understand that Mary was okay with going through with the "exam" without specifying the nature of the exam. Finally, it could be that Dr. Stimson was under the impression that he would be free to operate following the exam if he confirmed that it was a tumor. There is a danger of bringing Mary out of anesthesia and then putting her under again if she decides to proceed with the operation.

The scene, as described, is horrifying, and no positive spin could be placed on the man's actions. At best, he was trying to calm down a totally hysterical woman. His methods would usually be reserved for someone who needed chemical restraints. It wouldn't be for someone who was going for a procedure. This brings us to some pivotal points of discussion.

Let us suppose that Mary's account is accurate. It is incredibly horrifying. What on earth would compel people to behave in this way? It certainly appears to trample on Mary's right to make her own decisions about her body. Even in 1907, medical practice was normally thought to engage the patient's consent before surgery.

Let's continue with Mary's testimony. Mary awakened from surgery and did not recognize the place with strange faces surrounding her. She had difficulty talking following the operation, and, not surprisingly, no one spoke to her about the operation. Several days later, Mary said she realized Dr. Cottle was changing her abdominal dressing. He advised her not to talk, "to keep quiet, and I must not talk about the operation to him or the nurses, or anybody…I suffered more than I can tell… I was cut across the stomach from hip to hip. He said that Dr. Stimson—that I should have to ask Dr. Stimson, that he did not do it, and I should ask Dr. Stimson what was done to me" (para. 75).

It is precisely this testimony that makes me believe that Mary's operation was a mistake. It was either an intentional patronizing approach to her health, an unethical mistake, or a mistake in communication. Either way, it certainly seems like a cover-up.

Mary then asked to see Dr. Stimson, but he had left the hospital—not for the day—but no longer practiced there. According to her testimony, she repeatedly asked Dr. Cottle what had happened, but Cottle would only reply that she needed to talk to Dr. Stimson, who had performed the surgery.

As for the actual surgery, Mary suffered several terrible sequelae. First, one of the reasons she could not talk was the fact that her mouth was "torn to pieces inside" (para. 77). She couldn't swallow. She was given mouthwashes, but that did not seem to help her. Then she had pains in her arms and coldness and numbness in her left hand. She spoke to Dr. Cottle about it, seeking relief and help. "He said it did not amount to anything; it would pass away" (para. 78).

According to Mary, her plight, like her request not to have an operation, went unheeded, adding injury to injury to insult. Dr. Cottle refused to examine her hand even though she complained that her "hand was cold, and her fingers were blue." How did the doctor respond? "He laughed and said that I was imaginative. I suffered pain in that arm and hand. Increased pain from a few days after the operation up to the time it turned black" (para. 78).

Repeated requests for help were denied. She couldn't have her doctor attend to her because it broke the hospital rules. Imagine her feeling of helplessness, almost like being imprisoned in the hospital. Given the testimony so far, it would not be difficult to believe that there was a conspiracy happening where the staff knew that the physicians had done something wrong. They are now in the process of covering up, not letting outsiders in, and yet not responding to Mary's frequent requests for help.

Mary continued to suffer. She screamed all the time. She couldn't eat or sleep. The intern claimed he didn't know what was wrong with her hand, but her request for an expert went unheeded. The day she noticed her hand turning black, Dr. Cottle looked at the hand without a specific comment related to it. Instead, he commented on how he tried to get the hospital board to relent and bring in someone else, but they refused. In essence, while Mary's hand was falling off, his hands were tied.

They treated Mary as if she were a child or perhaps a "hysterical" woman unable to follow the slightest information. Not only was she not a person throughout this saga, she was almost non-existent to the eyes and ears of the hospital staff. Dismissed so easily.

The features of requiring the adult's consent have very few qualifications placed on them. The very idea is that we should be free to pursue our goals. Respecting those choices is a sort of prime directive. In the literature (for those interested in pursuing this), it is known as respect for the individual's autonomy. At first glance, most people agree with this but consider applying some restrictions when faced with certain situations. The nature of these restrictions yields some key concepts for further articulation.

The judge in this case (Cardozo) proclaimed that "every adult of sound mind has the right to do what he wants with his own body." There are only two categories of individuals precluded from having this right. Having the right requires something of others. In this case, we must respect the wishes of adult patients of sound mind when choosing what should happen with their bodies. By the way, it does not mean that we cannot respect the wishes of someone who is not of sound mind or an adult. We just don't *have* to respect those wishes.

At the time of Mary's case, women were not considered equals to men (at least by many men). Some of the "evidence" put forward was that women were too emotional and incapable of proper reasoning. This was due to their female organs. The last half of the 19th century saw the development of women's movements that tried to counter the notion that women were illogical creatures. At least they were no more illogical than men. This is important, as it is another way of expressing the relationship between autonomy and reason. Women were thought to be less rational, which would also play out in having the right to make decisions. Now I am not for a minute saying that this was expressly stated in this case, and Mary's competence was never part of the actual case. We shall get back to that later.

If Mary had told the staff not to remove her uterus, they violated her wishes. For the moment, let us take that as the truth. It is also clear that even if Mary said nothing, her values would contradict those of her physicians. They found that removing the ovaries was her best "medical" option. Indeed, she was still alive at the time of the case's appeal to the New York State Supreme Court. Yet she seemingly found it more important to be left totally intact. Is there a way of determining who is correct? We shall return to the "sound mind" aspect of the Cardozo decision.

If we try to use our decision-making models in a real-world example, we can see how difficult it is to use the expected value model. We will have to suppose that the medical staff will respect her wishes.

She is faced with the option of having the ether exam and conditionally approving the hysterectomy based on the visual inspection from the exam. She can also opt for the choice of having the exam and being awakened and told what the findings were. This would probably mean a full awakening; if she decided to proceed with the procedure, it would have to be later. This

92

would subject her to, in essence, two instances of being put under. She would be doubling her risks of death from the anesthesia and its other risks. The third option is to have the exam, even if it turned out poorly in terms of her prognosis, to live with the condition. Each option would then branch out and include the risks involved. The medical staff would have to relay the probabilities of death, brain injury, nausea, remaining pain in the abdomen, surgical error leading to death, cancer leading to death, and the length of times it would take for these to happen and their duration. A tall order for anyone.

I would imagine many of you would be like me, at least in this respect: I kind of narrowed down all these implications and branches to the pain and suffering that comes with the operation and the likelihood of my longevity, compared with the pain and suffering with the do-nothing approach and the likelihood of my longevity in that respect. Approximate timings of knowing when things get bad would be helpful. More than that, I probably cannot digest.

Mary must have felt that being left intact meant more to her than life itself. It does not appear to be an irrational thought. It seems to be one result that a sound mind would choose. A sound mind might also choose to have the surgery. In her case, her range of choices does not appear to include an entirely irrational one. The only questionable piece of Mary's thinking might be along the lines that she wanted an ether exam. She seems utterly opposed to having an operation, so it's unclear why she wanted the ether exam. I suppose it was to firm up a diagnosis.

Cardozo's decision left no doubt that patients have the right to choose to have a medical intervention or to refuse one. Mary had that right in that no one objected that she was not of a sound mind at the time she came in for medical treatment. She certainly met the criteria of being an adult. Nor does the range of her options seem to be irrational. The only way to disregard her wishes is to say she is not of sound mind or restrict her autonomy because she is not choosing the best option. Historically we do not know if the medical staff felt that she was a hysterical woman incapable of making a sound decision, or if she just was a woman who did not know what was best for herself. If either was the motivation for ignoring her wishes (assuming she did express those wishes), then that is morally wrong.

These actual cases relate back to my career in nursing and ethics consultations. Typically, they are messy. My bias is to assume that a patient is of a sound mind when confronted with these issues. I am also aware that patients may be diminished in their decision-making capacity. But it is rare that I would think they were so diminished that they couldn't make a rational decision. Confirming that they understood the information being presented and the alternatives would be a minimal criterion for me.

The following case really highlights another real situation that is quite dramatic. It gets to the heart of patients making choices that health care providers don't like.

Dax Cowart

Dax Cowart was, by all accounts, a truly handsome newly minted vet returning home from service in Vietnam. He had served as a pilot, a rodeo star, and a football player. One gets the picture of an active, energetic person. If what a person does is an indication of what they value, then adventure and accomplishment surely mark his life. The poignancy of his case is further and most artfully displayed in two videos recording his experiences. One was recorded by Robert White, a psychiatrist who was called in at one point to assess Dax's competency. Words on paper are not nearly as impactful as the images and sounds of the actual treatment. It isn't that the words used below cannot elicit, to some measure, the suffering of Dax. To evaluate Dax's competency, we cannot remain aloof throughout the evaluation process. Yes, for some parts, aloofness may be called for, but not all.

All of Dax's vibrant personality changed in 1973. He came home from Vietnam at the age of 25. Dax had wanted to gain employment as a pilot for an airline, but apparently, other returning pilots had made the jobs scarce. To make some money in the interim, he joined his father, a real estate developer, on a journey to look at some land for potential development. As they returned to the car, his father inserted the key into the ignition and turned it to the on position. The key turn closed the circuit and initiated a spark. The spark excited the propane gas, which had been leaked into the valley unbeknownst to the pair. A terrible explosion ensued. As Dax recalled the event, he saw the flames engulfing the entire area. He pushed open the car door, and initially, he saw only one area not swallowed by the fire. It had heavy underbrush, and he perceived that he would have to run through the flames. He took off down the road for a half mile. A passerby came to the scene, and Dax begged him to give him a gun so he could end it all.

That did not happen. It would be quite unfair, of course, to put that moral weight on the back of a Good Samaritan. The first ambulance arrived, and Dax directed them down to where his father lay. Dax couldn't stand his skin being touched. The emergency crew agreed to pick him up by his belt and put him into the ambulance. After some time, they put him in one ambulance and his father in the other. They were taken to a local emergency room ten miles away. There the staff decided they didn't have the resources to care for the two burn victims and sent them along in one ambulance to Parkland in Dallas. It was a 150-mile drive. Little did Dax know at the time that his father didn't make it.

There, at Parkland, Dr. Baxter oversaw his care. Dax had suffered a 65 percent deep burn to both eyes, ears, and hands. By his admission, Dr. Baxter had flippantly responded to Dax's repeated requests to be allowed to die. He felt initially that Dax wasn't serious. Up to that point, he was in the shock phase of the injury and was also on narcotics. Later, he felt that Dax was trying to manipulate the people around him to get them to do what he wanted them to do. Well, wouldn't you?

A pause here is most important. Dr. Baxter's responses are quite instructive. Being in shock and on narcotics is quite relevant to the competency issue—at least a temporary incompetency. But using the language of "manipulation" is quite interesting. Typically, the word has a pejorative connotation to it. Manipulating others feels like a form of coercion—getting people to do what they otherwise wouldn't. It is not straightforward. It doesn't always have to be that way. Like I manipulated the lever to get the machine to work. But it does get to the point of control. So even Dr. Baxter's description of Dax replays a certain narrative that Baxter has about Dax's behavior. Dr. Baxter's attitude is somewhat reminiscent of the attitude of the staff some 60 years earlier at Mary's hospital. Not acceding to her wishes and generally ignoring the complaints, and not interacting. The two cases feature different clothes and medical tools for treatment, but little progress in human interaction.

In Dax's case they immediately instituted burn treatment protocols, including frequently debriding the burn tissue using diluted bleach and the like. This involved immersions into tubs of liquid. Dax has described it as being like being burned in boiling oil or being skinned alive. In other words, to save him, he had to be tortured, as he framed it.

Physiologically the treatment was necessary to save his life. Our skin, when healthy, which was pretty much absent for him, is our protection against infection. Most microbes are too big to penetrate healthy skin, and the environment contains numerous bacteria and viruses. The treatment could increase his chance of survival from 20 percent to almost 100 percent. It was the pain of getting there that counted against the result.

The result wasn't all that promising either. The explosion and subsequent burns had removed one eye, blinded him in the other eye, and gnarled his fingers into his hands, fusing the skin together. His hearing was severely impaired. As a note, his name was Don at the time of the accident, and he changed it to Dax because he had trouble distinguishing the sound of "Dan" from other names. It would take numerous surgeries to get him to be functional. His appearance would permanently be scarred.

The video of him in the hospital receiving treatment isn't exactly a testimonial to a caring environment. The staff carries on conversations with rock music in the background. They talk to each other but not to him. His humanity is being ignored. Now, of course, these are snippets, and they may have spoken to him all the time, so we should not judge harshly that this is a great portrayal of the circumstances in that respect. But the pain he felt and the objectification of him as a patient is significant, both in the sense of being taken care of by the health care team and the passivity of his being. He lacked control over anything and everything. He was the recipient of activities and treatments, not an agent. This passivity is highlighted by his repeated attempts to stop these painful procedures.

The response of the medical team was anything but positive. His journey had him in two hospitals. The first was Parkland. He would be there for nearly eight months. His complaints were totally ignored, including obtaining some legal representation. The staff, no doubt, felt that his condition rendered him incompetent in the legal sense. Indeed, his physician there made it clear during a subsequent interview that patients during that interval post-injury are both heavily sedated on narcotics and are in shock. Just to get a sense of what it was like over that period, how he had his fingers amputated, his right eye removed, and his left eye sewn shut. During this time, he continually asked to be allowed to die.

His journey continued when he went to the Texas Institute for Research and Rehabilitation. Dax arrived there on March 12, 1974. Approximately three weeks into his treatment, one of the residents mentioned that his rehab would extend over several years. Upon hearing this, Dax begins refusing wound care. He well understood that this would eventually cause him to die. When that didn't happen quickly enough, he refused food and water. A meeting was held with his mother and the team, and they all agreed, including Dax, to transfer him to another burn specialty hospital.

He was then sent to Galveston's University of Texas medical research branch, where he ends up remaining for the next 14 months. During this time, Dax has multiple skin grafts, and the physician advises that he needs more surgeries to maximize his mobility and functionality. During that time, it appears that he tried to commit suicide by crawling out of bed and jumping through a window. Due to his lack of mobility, he was unable to commit suicide. At that point, psychiatric services were consulted. Doctor White recorded much of this information and was brought in to determine Dax's competency. Doctor White determined that Dax, indeed, was quite competent. He was rational and lucid. Even though he is deemed competent by a doctor while he still could not get discharged from the hospital or anyone to cooperate with assisted suicide, at this point, Dax's behavior shifts from cooperation with all the treatments in rehab to two refusals. Eventually, he is discharged to his home. Even there, he again has a suicide attempt, this time by walking in front of a truck. Later he tries to overdose on medication. It is not clear why these two attempts failed. Eventually, Dax got his law degree, practiced law, and married. Quite remarkable when you think about it.

Here is the real connection between competency and the models we have put forward in a more theoretical context. This is a useful case due to its intricacies as well as features that help highlight how ethical theories work (and how they don't). The idea that Dax is incompetent removes his right to decide. The staff could believe this for any number of reasons. In this case, what seems to have been professed is that he was willing to die, and that committing suicide is tantamount to being of an unsound mind. After all, the staff understood that they could save his life. It might have been different if his prognosis had been different. That is to say that he would die anyway. Under this approach, allowing him to die would not be considered suicide (a questionable stand, but we leave it for now). He was going to die with no hope for the future; in any case, that is not where this example stands. He could live, and any desire for suicide is inherently irrational.

It is hard to figure out how it is irrational. Don't forget that this is about competency, and the hospital staff want to claim that he cannot make a competent decision. It might be that it wasn't his conclusion that brought about this rejection of his claim. Or that he was not in a position to claim because the pain and the drugs made it impossible (or highly unlikely) to manage through a proper decision process. This is a more plausible attack on Dax's autonomy—that he wasn't competent not because of the alternative he wanted, but because he wasn't sufficiently in charge of his faculties to control his decision-making.

What evidence did the health care team have to make that assessment? Well, his pain was obvious, and we know that can make it difficult for a Think Two. As a counterpoint and a central point, I wish to make, the pain and its intensity and duration (as Bentham would have had it) are critical to the equation. Turning the complaint on its head, why aren't we saying that the staff is not competent to decide because they do not have the knowledge of the value (in this case, disvalue) of the experience? It is necessary because prudence dictates that we decide not only based on the journey's outcome, but the path to get there. As Dax has said, even though he ended up quite happy, it wasn't worth it. According to his later self, nothing could make up for what he endured.

To assess whether Dax was competent would require more details about him than we possess. Nevertheless, his pain is relevant in both a positive way (he can place a value on it) and in a negative way, as it is hard for him to assess the long-term future with probabilities and the like. The latter stays with the paternalists and the health care team in Dax's case.

The most plausible of the justifications for the paternalistic approach is that Dax is too distraught and in pain to be able to think things through. Of course, there are cases where people cannot make decisions, such as when they are drugged to the point of being hazy or unconscious.

His physician at Parkland expressed that he did initially disregard Dax's requests. He didn't believe Dax was serious. After approximately one year, they moved Dax to a rehabilitation facility, where he did agree to try to go through rehabilitation. He gave it a go for three weeks. It didn't go very well, at least from his point of view. He refused any further therapy. His physician then was Dr. Larson, who felt that Dax's refusal was unreasonable. After all, he had already invested so much in getting where he was. At that point, a psychiatric consult was requested to determine Dax's competency.

Dr. White was the psychiatrist called in to evaluate his competency in making decisions. As a historical side note, it is due to Dr. White that so much of this was documented. Dax spoke candidly with Dr. White. He relayed to him the frequent nightmares and the pain. If he were allowed to go home, he couldn't wait for the inevitable overwhelming infection to kill him. Dr. White found that there was nothing irrational about Dax's thought process. He was anything but delusional.

For us, this is critical. Different people can quite differently describe the desired state. He wanted to die. He wanted to be free of pain and torment. Even if you think the former is irrational, there is no question that the latter is quite rational. Desiring that kind of pain and torment might put one into the irrational category.

Eventually, Dax was allowed to make his own decision and fought his way through his rehabilitation. He was concerned with what kind of life he could lead. He eventually became a lawyer. He had several people and technologies assist him in studying, etc. Ten years after the incident, he won the first case he litigated for a total of 7.4 million dollars.

Now you might think after that that making him go through all of this proves the struggle was worth it. The ends justify the means. But according to Dax himself, that is not how he assesses it. He firmly believes that it wasn't worth it. His response is a mix of rights-based concerns (no one has a right to torture someone) and utilitarian considerations (nothing can ever make up for the pain I experienced).

Nevertheless, it is interesting to note that once he possessed the right to choose, he continued with therapy. The steps along the way all have their value. Every painful debriding subtracts from the value of a successful legal career.

Paternalism, Autonomy for Mary and Dax

Mary's case played a pivotal role in the legal and ethical history of informed consent in the US. It sets the standard of the characteristics that endow the patient with the right. An adult with a sound mind gets you into the club. The sound mind portion is quite vague. It was never questioned whether Mary was of a sound mind. A sound mind has been interpreted with a much lower bar than being able to perform an EV calculation. I remain unsure if some staff might have had a different opinion of her. Remembering the culture of the times, it would be reasonable to hypothesize that the staff would consider Mary to be hysterical. It was a hysterectomy they performed, and there was a belief that women were prone to hysteria due to their biology. If she were truly hysterical, then there would be a utilitarian reason to intervene. If she did not possess the decision-making capacity for making decisions or having a sound mind, then her right to make the decision does not exist. Acting in her best interests would not interfere with her rights.

The staff treated her poorly post operatively. They ignored her complaints of pain in her hand. It turned black due to poor blood supply. The legal transcript of the case is unclear as to the cause. It was quite painful, and she did cry out through the night. It was so disturbing that they moved her out of the ward to another area. The lack of care is quite upsetting. She was treated without any respect.

Assuming that she was of sound mind, as the court did, then the staff acted inappropriately. There was testimony that the physicians never heard her say that she did not want the operation. It is a suspicious claim, as the physician who documented that she consented in the chart never testified (McCullough et al 127). There are a few possibilities that may have happened. The first is that Mary recounted everything accurately. The staff lied about not hearing her objections. They continued to intervene over her stated wishes. Why would they do this?

They might think she would be better off with the surgery. They decided that once she was under and already taking the risk of an anesthesia incident, it made sense to perform the hysterectomy rather than get her permission and put her under again. After all, they might reason, surely, she will be better off having the cancer removed with the least amount of risk.

It is a utilitarian argument. The benefit is a longer life. The assumption is that everyone wants that no matter what. The reality is that male physicians believe that is what they would want. There is not really any room for other preference systems.

This leaves two alternatives to follow. Do what they did and run roughshod over her wishes or nudge her in the direction they think is a desired outcome. They most likely believed that the best course of action was to have the surgery and remove the cancer. They might be puzzled by her demand not to have surgery.

It is difficult today to understand why they didn't approach her and try to clarify her preference. It doesn't appear that anyone promoted the value of surgery. The lack of communication is stunning. It is interesting that the medical records from the hospital indicate a lack of communication among the staff, mentioning that the doctors performing the procedure were unaware of Mary's preferences (McCullough).

The communication of preferences is one of the elements critical to protecting patient autonomy and generating the best results.

One can wonder about the what-ifs here. What if a discussion took place, and Mary stated she wanted to live without stomach pain? Also, she did not want surgery. The fact is she cannot have both of these satisfied. An exploration of what her fears were about the operation would have been useful. Perhaps she would have been nudged in the direction of surgery by framing her options that favored surgical intervention. The framing is not wrong, but it is not neutral. A positive description of the surgery and its outcomes can be played against the danger of doing nothing and its consequences. There is a question about the ethics of nudging. Is it coercion? We will revisit this question of nudging in Chapter 6.

The case of Dax is another example of trampling over patient wishes while trying to do what is best. It really serves as a cautionary tale. The doctors, in this case, really thought Dax was not competent. If they could demonstrate he was not competent, then they would not be violating his autonomy. However, their belief that he was not competent appears to have been based on his preferences. There was no indication that he did not understand the consequences of his actions.

They knew many, or even most, patients go through stages after suffering such severe injuries. Statistically, they could estimate that Dax would change his mind about the treatments if he just held out a bit longer. It is as if they are ignoring the cost of traveling down a certain path. Dax cannot ignore it. This happens all too often when people talk about choices. They think of the outcomes as being immediate. The path to get to the desired outcome may tip the balance of value.

The physicians really were considering what seemed to be a reasonable argument. They have learned that most patients are depressed at this point in their recovery. They also know that most patients adjust to their condition as they improve. Based on data, patients reveal ways to accommodate their predicament that patients would not predict for themselves. If you were going to bet about what would most likely get the patient to the best outcome, then the statistics tell you to gamble on having Dax suffer now. A true paternalistic move on the notion that "We know better."

Both cases highlight the conflict between the self-determination of patients and what is best for them. The conflict stems from these two ethical principles we try to live by. It is time to explore them.

Chapter 5

Underlying Philosophy

Debate and Ethical Theories

I have avoided any deep philosophical discussion until this point. It's time to turn to the debates that underlie the two paradigms. The paramount debate in the physician-patient relationship centers on who gets to make the decision. We have been stipulating until this point that it will be the patient. We have shifted the focus from who should own the choice to how the information needs to flow regardless of who makes the decision. It is time to address the philosophical issues. We need to address the right to make the decision and who possesses that right.

There is an interplay between the philosophical foundations concerning rights and the paradigms of informed consent and shared decision-making. We have been simply assuming that patients have a right to make the decision. Certainly, that would bode well for the shared decision-making model. It is at least one way that the patient would participate in the activity. It might be that patients only need to select the alternative they want as their part in sharing. However, this is not what the proponents of shared decision-making have in mind. It is not the only piece of the process in which the patient participates. We've gone to some lengths to indicate that the patient also needs to share information back with the health care provider. The health care provider can then assimilate the preference order from the patient to filter what information might be relevant. Then the patient will receive this information and combine their preferences with their intensities (I like chocolate ten times more than I like a movie trip) to make at least a reasonable choice among the options. This would add a second piece of participation on the part of the patient.

We still have not established in any way that the patient needs to be the one performing the activity of making a choice, only that they are providing the value information. One could think of it in this manner: two pieces of information need to be fed into a decision-making piece of software. One is the medical information with the associated risks. The other is the preference order with intensities provided by the patient. All that is left to do is to take the raw pieces of meat and put them through the grinder of the software algorithms. You run the application, and the results come out for the stakeholders to follow. When the activity is framed this way, there is another component to be considered in the ethics of this situation, consisting of two different questions. One is who is capable enough to perform the sausage making. The other is who is the best at sausage making.

We have already come across the legal approach to this matter in the Schloendorff case. We can call this the threshold criteria for competency. Judge Cardozo expressed it as an adult with a sound mind. It was not expressed as an adult with the best mind. It is already leaning toward the patient having the right, and autonomy will rule the day. This is still neutral to either of our two paradigms.

The law establishes that patients get to make the call except under certain conditions. They do not have the right when they are too young (typically under 18 years of age or the age of majority) or too debilitated mentally. Now the law is not as concerned as we might be about why we should make these exceptions to the rule. Suffice it to say that how we think someone gets a right to do a particular activity plays an essential role. There must be some criteria separating those who do and those who don't. Any argument about who should make the call will ultimately lead us back to those criteria. Let's take a quick look at what philosophers have thought about this extensively and written about rights.

The right to make a decision can emanate from either a utilitarian theory of ethics or what is referred to as a deontological one. We have already become acquainted with the utilitarian account expressed by Jeremy Bentham. It turns out that this version of utilitarianism aligns with a paternalistic approach. For example, interventions for the patient are permitted when doing so will cause the greatest happiness for the greatest number of people. One can only hope that would include the patient. Typically, the health care professional estimates what should be done. They do not consider how the choice will affect other people and their happiness. Their concern is how to promote the best outcome for this patient. The HCP will most likely use their own set of preferences to populate the equations. We have seen that isn't the right way to do it. And many HCPs have made a conscious effort to discover patient preferences. Yet the use of their own values and preferences is still prominent.

This approach violates personal autonomy. Do utilitarians have a way of getting around this? The question about letting the physicians decide when a choice has to be made revolves around the consequences of allowing them to make that choice. A utilitarian would argue that letting Dax die is a bad outcome. It is an irreversible outcome. Forcing him to take the treatments, while regrettable in terms of his emotional response at the time, is outweighed by the extension of his life and what he later was able to do.

There is another way that at least some utilitarians have modified their approach or adopted a different approach. It still relies on the consequences, as does the method outlined above. You can take note of the fact that the above method evaluates the consequences of one particular action. This is known as act utilitarianism. Philosophers are quite clever, you know. To manage situations that seem to require a rule and freedom and other intuitions, a second-order utilitarianism has been developed. It is called rule utilitarianism. You may have guessed that this approach evaluates some rule instead of evaluating an act. The rule will be evaluated on whether it creates the most happiness for the stakeholders. In our case, the outcomes would be from a rule which allows patients to make their own decisions. The idea is that the outcomes are better than when you let the HCP make the decision. The hypothesis would be that intervening occasionally would create distrust between physicians and patients and a lack of compliance. Together, these two would result in worse outcomes than letting patients make their own decisions, even though some patients will make bad ones.

The other set of theories is known as deontological theories. The word "deontology" comes from the Greek "deon," which means duty. The other part of the word relates to the Greek term "logos." Logos means the study of or the science of something. It is an approach that uses laws or maxims to guide our behavior.

A well-known example would be, "one should always keep their promises." It doesn't give an excuse for deviating from the rule. It doesn't matter if it leads to adverse consequences. The principle of respecting a patient's autonomy relies on some laws within ethics about respecting other persons. Immanuel Kant was a great proponent of the deontological theory. He put together a two-level approach. He developed clever criteria to assess whether a maxim qualifies as a moral law, patterned after physical laws. They would need to be universally applicable to all persons in similar circumstances. One example would be a maxim about keeping promises. Should all promises be kept? Kant would answer yes. To allow exceptions would make the activity of promising unsustainable. Well, at least, so he would argue.

The choice of which action to take would be governed by a maxim generated by the person. Such a maxim might be, "Do unto others as you would want them to do unto you"—a very familiar one. The maxim is then tested by a formulation of what he called the Categorical Imperative. There were five formulations of these, by my count. The one closest to the Golden Rule would be this one: "Act so that you treat humanity, whether in your own person or in that of another, always as an end and never as a means only" (Kant p .47). Deontologists often find a feature or characteristic of an action and then make the action into a rule to be followed.

Kant had an interesting take on the idea of a person. In the moral realm, it is somebody who can freely make choices. They are not swayed by physical emotions, and they're capable of following rules. Obligations are only required for people who can follow rules. A Kantian view would easily support the idea that only those who can rationally make maxims are free people.

An example would be that I understand what is meant by making a promise. If I engage in that kind of activity, I will myself to make sure I keep my promises. It differs from keeping a promise as a result of somebody pointing a gun at your head and coercing you. It is done of your own free will, according to Kant. Kant's arguments for this approach are confusing for sure, and they ultimately fail. Grounding ethical theories is extremely hard to do. Grounding them successfully is even harder, for sure. Those arguments go well beyond the scope of this book. My many years of teaching ethics in health care have allowed me to see that most of us align with both deontological and utilitarian justifications for what is the right thing to do. Naturally, the answer we want comes immediately to mind, and we look for the ethical theory that supports it. We don't start from the theory we believe in and then discover what action should be supported.

The deontological approach aligns well with respect for autonomy. You can just take Cardozo's proclamation and say that anyone who is an adult with a sound mind has the two characteristics required for being a person in Kant's sense. Persons deserve respect for their decisions. Controlling your destiny entails making your own decisions, not someone else making those decisions for you. It is necessary to have the ability, yet having the ability is not enough. You need the opportunity and support to do it.

There are other utilitarian theories and deontological accounts within each camp. The primary difference between the utilitarian and deontological theory types is that utilitarian theories rest on consequences, and ontological theories do not.

Looking at the two ethical alternatives, the utilitarian theory provides the following arguments in favor of the physician decision-maker. The decisions will more likely lead to better results either because of a better understanding of the medical situation and/or how other patients have fared with various decisions. The principle being followed is that of beneficence—doing what is good. You probably have noticed that we don't really think of rights in terms of beneficence. The consequences of the act do not play a role in their rightness or wrongness. You have a right to make harmful decisions, as it were. That doesn't mean you want to, of course. This approach will most easily follow deontology. Let us see if there is any pull-through from the deontological approach to informed consent and shared decision-making paradigms.

The principle here is autonomy. As mentioned above, not every possible decision-maker has the right. Rights under this sort of ethics are conferred on those who possess certain qualities. According to the Schloendorff court, if you are an adult with a sound mind, you get this right. Let's see if we can make some sense of this.

The right to perform this act really requires competency in exercising the right. Consider how silly it sounds to say you have the right to levitate in the air or some other impossible feat. It isn't that the statement is true or false. The statement really doesn't make much sense. The nature of having a right is that under some sort of standard circumstances, you can exercise the right. I can hear you say, "But what if I am not given the opportunity?" Well, that should be eliminated as a test case because we are clearly talking about standard circumstances which must include the opportunity. Some of the confusion around this in conversation with others stems from the idea of being able to perform an action. The act here involves decision-making, and it requires a sound mind to be able to make good decisions. This sounds reasonable. If this characteristic of the patient is present, then they get the prize. If not, someone else must make the decision and pass the test of having a sound mind.

The sound mind requirement helps in one regard. It makes it more likely that a good decision will be made. It begs the question of how sound the mind must be, though.

The deontological approach does not solely rely on consequences to determine the right to decide. However, competent decision-making ability should lead to acceptable consequences if performed under the right conditions.

Utilitarians have several responses to these approaches. So, one might respond that even though patients are not best equipped to make the decisions, the fact that they get to make the decision makes them happier. This needs to be part of the utilitarian equation. This maneuver is called rule utilitarianism. The rule is judged rather than just the assessment of one act. It is an acknowledgment that a particular case may end up with bad consequences, but if you stick to the rule, you will end up with good consequences overall. Sometimes patients choose a less-than-optimal or good alternative for themselves. Even so, that one bad outcome will be greatly outweighed by the satisfaction patients will have by deciding for themselves. The process will provide more patient satisfaction. The fact that patients are more compliant when they are involved is an indication that there are some positive outcomes from letting them participate in decision-making (Deniz 1).

Let me illustrate this point. John must decide between getting surgery to remove a clot or a medical intervention. The physicians have pointed out the advantages and disadvantages of each approach. John is not thrilled with either route. Instead, John chooses not to go down either road and refuses treatment. This choice increases his likelihood of death astronomically. For the sake of argument, let us say that John throws the clot and has a stroke. The act utilitarian approach would say physicians should have intervened and forced one of the therapies on John. He would not have had a stroke, most likely.

The rule utilitarian rule would say letting people make their own decisions is a far better way of promoting happiness than intervening on the odd occasion. Not only does one contend with John's unhappiness of being forced to do what he doesn't want to do, you need to multiply those times everyone else's unhappiness when it happens to them. They will claim that when you do the math, you have better outcomes than when you force treatment. Factors that may sway toward this result include patients' reluctance to seek medical care because they feel they will be coerced into treatment. Consequently, more patients will not seek care. They will be sicker as a result.

The deontological approach looks at some features of the action to determine if the action is right. We are not as interested in the "right" action but who has the right to perform the action. For this analysis, we are drawn to some features of the agent. Immanuel Kant historically puts forth a rather seminal way to approach the topic. Persons are always to be treated as an end and never merely as a means. In other words, I need to be seen and treated as the author of my goals and endeavors. This fits more easily into this discussion.

The pivotal issue for this approach is that Kant believes that the rights a person has and our obligation to expect that right is connected to them being a person. The definition of an autonomous person is someone rational and capable of giving and taking in reasons for choices. This is quite close to the Schloendorff case pronouncement that those of adult years and sound mind have the right to make their own choices. They deserve to be treated with respect.

The upshot is that there are good reasons from either ethical approach to support the patient's decision-making preference. Both approaches make the intuitive requirements that whoever is making the decision needs to be able to take in information and assess it. In one case, it leads to better results than in the other because that is what it means to be free and autonomous. It also conforms to the major legal decisions about restrictions on the right and links the right to the decision-making process.

So, who wins here? Both camps would agree on the adult piece of the equation. At what age someone is an adult is somewhat vague and changes with time. The basic notion, as the Goldilocks tale would indicate, is that experience plays a role in the endeavor to make a good decision. Figuring out the medical facts does not take experience. Child prodigies graduating from medical school at an extremely early age can calculate the best course of action given their desired outcome. In fact, there are algorithms that tell you what courses of action are most likely to lead to the outcomes of choice. Selecting the outcomes of choice is the tricky part. Which of the many outcomes is preferable, given the journey to that outcome?

If we started looking at preference selection, including the journey to get there, I believe there would be less confusion. My view is that the choices are made to look more like a gambling scenario where you get your cost upfront and the outcome right away. There are not a lot of steps in between. The reality is that the outcomes are not instantaneous following the initiation of treatment. Typically, there are a number of steps between the initial treatment and the final outcome. The expected value model makes us calculate each intermediate step to put it into the equation for how good or bad that journey is.

Moving beyond the question of how we come up with values is the very interesting problem of how having a sound mind comes into play. I am going to give a bit of leeway here in the discussion and allow for the idea of competency to be something above that required by law. I understand that the legal definition of competency only requires the patient to understand the options. The patient needs to be awake when making the decision. They need to be under no duress from the staff. Of course, this doesn't consider a living will type situation. The patient may be comatose when a decision must be made. This just moves the criteria back to when the living will was created. During the creation of the living will, the patient will still have to meet the criteria of having a sound mind at the time. During the prior time, they must be under no duress from other sources such as other medical care providers. A living will follows some of the same rules as a typical will.

The reason for upping the ante here is that we would like to support patient autonomy and good decision-making. That is the goal of whatever paradigm we are choosing, whether it be informed consent or shared decision-making. The ethical point of view may require more because we need to figure out how competent decision-making relates to being a person. This is decidedly a deontological approach. We are going to look at a characteristic of human beings to determine if that characteristic is sufficient to confer personhood on them. In other words, if they are competent, then they are a person.

The philosophical argument for this falls along these lines. When a person makes rational decisions and is competent at it, then they are behaving in a free and independent manner. They are not succumbing to external pressures and forces. It is through their rational thought that they come to their choice rather than being forced to do so solely based on emotions, chemical imbalances, and other physical causes. The rational thought process brings human beings out of the causal nexus.

This type of argument also reaches back into the history of philosophy. Once again, Immanuel Kant says something similar to this. It is quite an interesting approach. If you believe in causation, how can you say you're free to make these choices? Rational thought doesn't fall under the causal nexus of physics, so the argument goes.

A way of illustrating this is to consider when a person is drugged compared to when they are not. While under the influence of drugs or alcohol, they do not typically make good decisions. The effects of the chemicals drive their thought process. People are more susceptible to their emotions driving their decisions. They don't think forward into the future to project outcomes that may occur. Often, they lack an understanding, in the moment, of their limitations. So once the substances have been ingested, people are more or less at the mercy of the chemical byproducts. That puts their decision-making apparatus right in the middle of a causal chain. That chain is certainly a physical one. Once this has happened, it is questionable whether they are freely making a decision.

If, however, the person has not ingested any of these products, then their decisions are solely based on the information they have and their decision-making abilities. Crudely and perhaps with some naivete, the thought is that kind of thinking lies outside a physical causal nexus. It is what some people would say is one way of exercising your free will.

This brings up another interesting point. One of the meanings of a free choice is that no external party is coercing you. They haven't drugged you. They haven't pointed a gun at your head. It doesn't mean you are free from your physiological brain mechanisms. No one would argue that this is a necessary condition for being free. It is also a less controversial approach to the concept of freedom.

Although quite interesting for the concept of freedom, the approach does nothing to help us understand the concept of a sound mind. Admittedly, it was never introduced to perform that task. There are certainly other problems with it. It is easy to understand external coercion by others. It is less easy to see internal components playing a role.

Is there a way to figure out what constitutes sound mind in this context? We can get back to whether that confers personhood on an individual later. The approach we will take is to understand a sound mind, not as a passive status. It involves an activity, in our case, which is decision-making. Decision-making goes beyond purely understanding information. At the end of the day, you're going to make a choice, and you want to make a choice that will get you to your preferred outcomes. That is putting you more in control. Autonomy means self-control. One thing we know at this point is that the decision-making process involves evaluating outcomes in terms of personal preferences and combining that with likelihoods. This, in turn, requires a knowledge of personal preferences in terms of their intensity. One needs to be able to compare preferences from different dimensions. These characteristics are neutral toward whether it is the physician or the patient who makes the decision. Some of that conclusion will be based on which philosophical theory you adopt. Other parts of that decision (whether it's the physician or the patient who should make the decision) are based on the criteria for competency. There are two ways to draw judgment. The first is that the patient is the default chooser so long as they meet the minimum criteria for competency. A different approach is to select the decision-maker who is more competent.

We need to figure out what it means to be a competent decision-maker before we can rightfully answer the question of who gets to do it.

When we say that a person is competent at doing something, then we know they can do it. It is time to investigate the meaning of the word "can."

The Can of Competency

What does it mean to say that a person can do something? This statement has a variety of meanings. In the Encyclopedia of Philosophy, Bruce Aune conveniently listed the various meanings of "can." The list includes the following:

The "can" of right
The "can" of inclination or probability
The "can" of opportunity
The "can" of possibility
The "can" of ability

It is highly likely that one of these is the meaning associated with competency. In turn, let us look at these candidates and see which is the best choice. It will involve capturing the idea that competency does not involve luck. It should allow someone to be considered competent even if they lack the opportunity to display it. When you are not given information about procedural risks, you are deprived of the opportunity to demonstrate your competency in decision-making. The idea of success needs to be incorporated somehow, even if it isn't in the actual circumstances. As we might be deprived of the opportunity to exercise our competent decision-making, we can imagine a world with the opportunity where we would be successful.

The "can" of right is the "can" of permission and is interchangeable with the term "may." One example is: "You can borrow five dollars."

This can of permission is eliminated as a possible candidate for the following reason. In the medical context, it would be possible to give a person permission to make the decision at hand even if that person were not competent. Thus "the person can make the decision," where we mean that the person has permission to make the decision, tells us nothing of the person's competency for making a decision.

Likewise, the "can" of inclination can be eliminated. One example of this sense would be, "I was so hungry, I could eat a horse." This sentence expresses a degree of hunger and does not really address itself to the competency of the person to perform the act.

The "can" of opportunity is expressed in the following: "He could have played tennis if he had known how." Obviously, this sentence expresses a lack of competency rather than a possession of it. It, too, will be eliminated as a potential candidate. However, it should be noted that the concept of "opportunity" will play a role in the concept of "competency."

According to the list of possibilities, there remain two. The competitors are the "can" of possibility and the "can" of ability. In what follows, I intend to show that the possibility sense is not the appropriate sense of "can" for explicating the concept of competency.

Using the methodology previously employed, we start with the statement, "It is possible for the person to make a decision." Is this enough to explicate the sentence "the person is competent to make a decision"? It is not, as the following makes clear.

There are at least two ways in which the person can accomplish the task of doing an activity. The person can be competent in performing the task, or the person can be lucky and get it done. One example would be throwing snake eyes in a game of dice. It is a game of chance. I might throw the pair, and they'll each come up a one. Yet, I wouldn't claim I am competent at throwing snake eyes. Better yet, take the example of shooting an arrow toward a target 50 yards away.

I have never drawn an arrow with a bow, and I'm unlikely to hit the target. After much practice, I get closer, but I never hit the target, much less the bull's-eye. On one occasion, I draw back the string and unleash the arrow, and it's heading way off target. A gust of wind (a major actor in the examples surrounding abilities) comes along and blows my arrow right toward the bull's-eye. This would hardly be an example of a competent archer. In both cases, it was possible for the person to perform the task, but they were not competent. Hence, the "can" of possibility will not serve us well in an analysis of competency.

This leaves us with the "can" of ability as the explicating concept. However, there are two ways of unpacking the "can" of ability. This is reflected by the two phrases "being able to" and "having the ability to." The former seems to be linked closely with the "can" of possibility. This is made clear by looking at the examples below, which I draw from the work of Locke (1974 pp1-2).

Someone may have the ability to play tennis and hit the ball in bounds. On a particular occasion, the player may lack the opportunity or hit out of bounds. Having the ability to play tennis does not require perfection on every stroke.

On other occasions, someone may not have an ability but be able to succeed because they get lucky, like hitting the bull's-eye.

One can also not have the ability while still successfully performing the task, as when a mother saves her child pinned by a car and lifts the vehicle and frees her child. She is able to do it—it is possible. On the other hand, she cannot lift cars under any other circumstances.

The three types of distinctions imply that the two senses are not reducible to one another. One may be able to do something without having the ability to do it. This shows us that "being able to" is not reducible to "having an ability." Similarly, one may have the ability to do something without being able to do it. This shows that "having an ability" is not reducible to "being able to."

The "being able to" sense seems closely linked to the "can" of possibility. If it is possible for a person to do an activity, then the person is able to do it. If the person is able to do it, then it must, in some sense, be possible for the person to do it.

We are still left with the problem of explicating the concept of competency.

How does all of this help? The "being able" sense will fail here just as the "can" of possibility did. As the second distinction indicates, one is able to do things through luck, and, of course, this will not do as an explanation of competency. Conversely, as in the first example, one could be competent but unable to make a prudent decision because one is not properly informed of the risks involved. They lack the opportunity.

Not surprisingly, the concept of ability remains the only alternative. There are some problems with this as well.

A man might have to climb a ladder up to a fourth rung to change a light bulb. Indeed, he has shown the ability to climb one rung, even four times in a row. In any obvious sense, he has the opportunity. But he is so petrified by fear that he cannot bring himself even to attempt to reach the height of the fourth rung, though he would succeed if he were to try. Despite having both the ability and the opportunity, he is unable to do it.

One interesting feature of this example is how it parallels a relevant type of medical situation. Sometimes patients are fearful. Many people believe that these fears prevent patients from being able to make decisions. These patients might be considered incompetent, though they would still possess the ability to make decisions.

Some people might try to avoid this result in the example by questioning whether this man really had the ability in question. After all, the action is described as climbing to the top of the ladder, and clearly, this man cannot do that now or at any other time. He does not possess that ability. A similar move could be made in the medical example, and it would end up that the patient was not competent and did not have the ability.

I am extremely uncomfortable with this maneuver, which amounts to specifying conditions to a point where the person does not have the ability in question. It does seem to me that the man in the example has the ability but cannot bring himself to exercise it. If we accepted the position that he doesn't have the ability, then for each different context of climbing, we would require a different climbing ability. Indeed, we would all have an infinite number of climbing abilities. Although this remains a possible solution, it seems to me to be too awkward and ad hoc.

A better analysis of the ladder example is to agree that the man has the ability to climb up the steps of the ladder. What he lacks is the ability to overcome his fear, which will be necessary to exercise his climbing ability.

Perhaps an example from the world of sports will help illustrate the point. It is a well-known fact among athletes that the players on the professional tennis tour hit the ball equally well in practice. The difference in their stroking abilities is minimal. Yet, when they play in tournaments, most players don't play quite as well. They "tense up" or "choke." Psychologically, they lack the ability to relax and concentrate under pressure. They haven't lost the ability to stroke the ball well; they just don't have the psychological ability to exercise it during a match. This also helps to explain why some players appear to have "all the ability in the world" but never "put it together" or can't get up for the contest and, therefore, don't play well. These athletes do have the ability to perform well but don't have the ability to exercise that ability.

Applying these results to the medical context, we find that competency is a bit more complicated than being a simple ability. I think that we would all agree that if people were so possessed by fear that they couldn't attempt to think through the decision, we would say that they were not competent. Of course, if they tried, they would succeed (keeping the examples parallel). They have the ability to make the proper decision but are unable to exercise that ability. And they are unable to exercise that ability because they lack the ability to overcome the fear. They are not competent.

We can, and should, distinguish this medical example from one where patients cannot decide prudently because they lack the information. Here the patients are unable to exercise their abilities as well, but not because of a lack of ability. Basically, these people lack the opportunity. They still may be very competent.

Finally, there will be cases where the patients simply lack the ability, as in cases of coma or severe retardation. These patients will be considered incompetent.

We can give a formal definition of competency. These examples led me to make the following analysis of competency: A patient is competent in making decisions if and only if the patient's constitution and history are such that if the patient were to attempt to make a decision where the standard conditions for making decisions obtain, then the patient, by the patient's own intentional actions caused by the patient's constitution and history, would succeed in making good decisions an appropriate percentage of the time. I know what you're thinking. This is supposed to be the easy philosophical approach. It is the standard way academic philosophy would approach giving a definition. Let's take a moment and break this down.

Intuitively we think of somebody as being competent through the exercise of their own capacities and functionalities. They were either born with the competency or acquired it through diligent practice and exercise. This is why we have placed the patient's constitution and history into the definition.

We want the action to be intentional. Suppose four tennis players are playing a doubles match. One of the players is at the net. He is looking up at the sky because he doesn't pay attention very well to the match. The opponents hit a crosscourt shot that hits his racquet while he gazes at the clouds. The ball ricochets back over the net for a winning shot. Our net player had no intention of hitting that ball when it came across the net. We wouldn't know if he is a competent volleyer because that return was unintentional and not a result of his abilities.

The definition given above is dependent on the notion of success. In fact, would you say someone is competent at a particular activity when they succeed a certain percentage of the time? Keeping with the sports analogies, a baseball player who gets hits only 30 percent of the time is considered outstanding. The more difficult the activity, the lower the percentages will be. At the other end of the spectrum would be signing your name without making a spelling error. Here we would expect a 100 percent success rate. At least, I would.

The trickiest piece of this is the hypothetical world that would constitute standard conditions. I introduced this in my PhD thesis back in the 1980s. It was meant to manage several fairly deep philosophical objections. Those objections were based on miraculous gusts of wind, as in the archer example. Philosophers love to create artificial conditions to upend definitions. It seems to me that we have some paradigm in mind for the various activities we engage in. In sports, they do not typically include miraculous gusts of wind. Accounting for predictable meteorological elements may be part of being a competent tennis player for sure. By definition, you cannot account for a miraculous gust of wind. If that happened all the time, it would be impossible to be successful except through luck.

Let's apply this to decision-making, which is the point of delving into this. How would we assess a person's competency, be it a patient or health care provider, in making these decisions? The standard conditions for making decisions would be that information is provided by yourself and another source. Value comparison across different dimensions will occur in these standard conditions. The decision-maker must have a way of ordering preferences and comparing intensities across dimensions. One example would be comparing increased functionality against the experience of increased pleasure. The choice situation will not involve any coercion. The question will be if the decision-maker has given evidence of being successful under those conditions. The conditions here are being presented with medical alternatives.

I suggest that a person is a competent decision-maker if they have previously demonstrated the ability to make decisions that consider information relevant to their priorities. They will have demonstrated that they can project into the future and imagine what it would be like to live with the consequences. They have successfully performed these activities in the medical context or some other important situation. The question remains: What success rate are we looking for here?

The success rate can be seen as high when we make important decisions if the criterion for success is fairly low. What I mean by this is that a successful decision doesn't have to lead to the optimal result. It is more like horseshoes. Getting close counts. I cannot at this time offer a quantitative percentage for success in this paradigmatic world. It is more like the idea that success is picking an option that makes sense for the individual. That is, it does align with some set of values and preferences of the patient.

Look at the case of Dax as an example. He lived in an environment with a future that was at odds with his past. He would no longer be handsome or athletic. His estimate would be that he suffered a severe loss, which surely seems accurate. He is suffering through the experience of keeping his wounds clean through the excruciatingly painful debriding process. I mean, outside of the long chance of getting better, there appears to be nothing irrational about ending his life. Mind you, if he had been a devoutly religious person and his religion prohibited ending his life, then it might not be the right choice. It would not satisfy his professed goal.

The case of Mary Schloendorff is a little bit more complicated. Besides the facts being a little harder to sift and sort, she seemed to be in possession of her faculties, and she decided to leave the West Coast after the earthquake. She sought medical care for the pains in her stomach. She thought she understood what would happen to her, and when she didn't fully comprehend what was going on, she asked legitimate questions. These questions related to her immediate future and whether she was having surgery.

Mary and Dax both successfully did what a competent decision-maker would do. They asked questions that were related to reality. The questions were related to their specific goals. Both seemed to be worried about their future experiences and functionality. We know less about Mary, her desire for her future, and what it would mean after a hysterectomy. One certainly gets the sense that it was self-defining for her. Perhaps she even valued it more than life itself. Did she accurately judge her future experience?

It would be easier to detail this if we had consistent preferences over time, but unfortunately, we do not. Take the case of Dax. Choosing not to have the treatment and end his life seems quite rational because he is being "tortured." It is also reasonable for someone in his situation to opt for getting treatment and wanting to live. Neither choice is irrational, with the result being an incompetent patient. It really depends on whether the choice is more likely to fit within their preference system than some absolute standard. It is incumbent on the health care team to elicit from the patient their preferences. Shared decision-making proponents have done studies to help with values clarification for patients. I would suggest that success is arriving at the decision most likely lead to satisfaction with the patient's expressed preferences and values.

It might be easier to see the point by looking at its opposite. What would a failure look like? The patient goes through values clarification in a situation similar to Dax. They say they want to live no matter how much pain they suffer. Then when they come to the baths, they say "I just don't want to do this, let me die." The staff points out that by not doing this, the patient will die and thus not be achieving the goal they had originally professed.

Now it is not unreasonable for a person to want two things, but they can't have both. The question here would be whether the patient understands this impossibility and can choose only one. If they do not understand this dilemma as being a dilemma, then I would question their competency. On the other hand, most patients understand this conceptual dilemma, and they're just expressing their reluctance to go through the pain and their desire to live. It is a tough choice. Competent decision-makers with those values would recognize this as a dilemma. Either choice, electing treatment or denying treatment, would be rational. One could hear somebody say, "I am willing to go through the pain if I can restore functionality in my life and be like Dax." Assume they go through the procedures and go on to live. However, they do not gain the functionality that Dax obtained. They guessed wrong about future events. They would have recognized (this is all hypothetical) that the future is uncertain. They undertook the risk. In a world of uncertainty, a failed objective is not a sign of a failed process.

Some people would say that under the circumstances choosing to be allowed to die (refusing treatment) is rational for them. They don't want the painful process to continue even if they know it will end in 26 months. Once you have had the pain, it is easier to calibrate how bad it feels.

There are a lot of practical issues in determining this ethical competency. It needs to be rather quick and simple, if possible. As a health care provider, you will not know this person's decision history. You will be confronted with their present situation for the most part. You're most likely to allow that they are competent decision-makers if they successfully display typical everyday decision-making activities. They display an understanding of the information if tested. They can coherently talk about themselves. They can remember events from the morning of that day. They can tell you what they want and what they don't want. They can project into the future. They don't order a roast beef sandwich for lunch and then tell you they don't eat meat.

The shared decision-making paradigm allows for this kind of give-and-take far more than the informed consent paradigm. The values clarification piece helps the patient determine what they might really want. More to the point, they may be able to create a crude hierarchy of preferential outcomes. The health care provider, in turn, may understand the journeys that will take the patient to each of those outcomes and their likelihoods. Together they can discuss some level of detail about these different journeys. Where does that journey end?

My "Future Self"

At first glance, the concept of a successful outcome does not appear to be all that complicated. If we continue, as I think we should, with the idea that the patient should make his or her own choices, then they should evaluate the outcomes. After all, they are the ones that place value on the outcomes projected in the first place. This fact allows for some interesting challenges. Let me introduce you to another behavioral economics experiment that relates quite a bit to the journey.

One series of experiments subjected the participants to small shocks of varying intensities over time. If you add it up, their immediate response is at each interval; you would get a value for each shock and the pain experienced at the time, say on a scale of one to ten. Suppose during the sequence, the first shock was a three, the second a five, and the third a two. The total amount of pain would be $3+5+2 = 10$. When looking in hindsight, you do not have to supply probabilities since the events happened.

This brings another factor into our deliberations. Will I have the same preferences when I receive the first shock as when I receive the second? How about the third? The closer these events happen to the journey's beginning, the less likely I will shift my evaluations.

As it turns out, we do not value the journey the same way after it is completed. Instead, it is the last experience that outweighs all the prior experiences. In our example, the last shock was a two. We would be inclined to say that we averaged about a two on a one to ten scale. In essence, it impacts how we feel about the entire experience. The average is 3.3 if each instance has an equal say.

This brings up a very tough challenge yet to be met. We have defined competency to make decisions as being related to a success rate. We are having issues defining what that rate would be, but there is a further issue: It is very hard to determine what is a success. I would say that we normally look at the results of our decisions and turn them into either good or bad. We can only do this in hindsight. Hindsight would be a future self looking back on the events leading up to that point in the future.

It is critical to understand how we will evaluate the success or failure of the choices and the process—getting back to the beginning of this work, the major critique of the paradigm of informed consent was that patients were not given the information they needed nor how they needed it. That failure is easy to chalk up. Physicians and health care providers didn't know what would be relevant for patients. When reviewing studies done for shared decision-making and some of its successes, patient comprehension of the information is included. This, of course, is one of the necessary pieces of the exchange that has to occur. You can also mark off patient satisfaction with the interaction. It certainly is improved in a shared decision-making context, as it is unclear to me whether this is an important criterion for success. It is, of course, on its own a good thing. It may even be instrumental in another component, which is patient compliance with the agreed-upon therapy. This compliance is important from their medical point of view, at the very least. It also means that if the patient has chosen wisely, they are more likely to achieve their goals sooner rather than later.

The fact is that my future self and my present self may dispute whether, in fact, I made the right choice. It is the present self that must make the decision because we might not know what our future self would say. When I was twenty-five, I had many ideas about what was best for me. As life goes along, I have discovered many surprising things about those ideas. There are some things I thought I would not enjoy but have found otherwise. We might say let us bless the utilitarians, for they would enjoy all these positive outcomes.

The nut that is tough to crack concerns which self should evaluate success, and what natural approaches we need to just look at what we do. The answer will depend upon the question we're asking about success. One formulation was that it was a good decision, given the circumstances under which it was made. I tend to think this is the question of interest here. We can return to nine blue balls in an urn versus one red ball. I place a wager that a blue ball will be pulled. A red ball is pulled. Was my decision a good decision? At the time, it was when I made it. I had a much better chance of having a positive outcome. As luck would have it, didn't work out that way.

Even though I made a rational and good decision, the outcome was not successful. The evaluation of the outcome as being a success appears not to be inexorably linked to the rationality involved at the decision stage. We would judge the competency of the decision-maker according to whether they followed certain expected processes. It is only when these processes continually miss the mark that we may question them. So once again, when we miss the mark, we are admitting to failure. We still must gauge whether an outcome was successful.

This brings us full circle back to the shock problem. Sorting this out, it's a little bit complex. We may have correctly identified at each time point the value we place on the shock (the value here would, of course, be a negative one). We also know that whatever decision-making model we employ requires us to evaluate the steps along the way. One item that we haven't seen is a change in how we evaluate those steps on the journey. Indeed, it is important that we pay attention to our future self. Not only are we predicting what events will occur, but when we are placing value on those events, it is through our present preferences. Should we pay attention to our future self?

This conceptual difficulty is pretty thorny. Let us lay it out. We have the point in time where the decision will be made. Let us call this time T1. The decision-maker will have certain values and preferences at that time. The decision-maker will have to predict what events are likely to happen and the value and intensities of those possible outcomes. They will have to compare those outcomes across those dimensions, most likely. Often this is where we end our analysis. Now we can see that there are other time points in the future to be considered.

There are time points T2 and T3 as well. At each of these time points, we may have quite a different evaluation of any of the outcomes. I suspect that if T1, T2, and T3 are all close together in time, we would not expect drastic changes in evaluating the pain. On the other hand, if we space these five years apart, we would not be surprised if the same level of electricity yields a different outcome.

For example, someone in their late teens is given certain options about work. They enjoy work and find no problem with staying late. They do not have significant others in their life, perhaps. Work is their satisfaction. They are on a path to career advancement. It's a fairly good thing.

Now let us suppose that our protagonist has children (assume the children are distant cousins who are now his responsibility). At the time of receiving this new responsibility, there is a certain resentment of foiling a person's desires. He may have made choices earlier in his career where life satisfaction was solely related to career advancement. Lo and behold, our hero really enjoys parenting. So even though he would not have chosen this and reluctantly accepted the responsibility, he now feels it is more important and rewarding to be a parent. People can change their values and preferences over time. Perhaps this needs to be incorporated into the shared decision-making paradigm.

You may remember that it was somewhat difficult to know when to stop calculating in the expected value model. That problem is back again. It isn't surprising since this is a consequentialist model that we're supplying. It also appears that we need to be cognizant of our future dispositions as human beings. Even if we can produce them, as in the electric shock example, we must decide how to evaluate the journey. Making evaluations across the dimensions, it's like getting different voters' opinions. If you're someone who isn't going to change much over time, this becomes less of an issue. If you are a person who is going to change, then you produce these paradoxes in collecting votes.

This can be found in Appendix B, with a rather lengthy treatment using the decathlon to combine disparate utility functions. My view, without a substantial philosophical rigor behind it, is that we judge what we would like when the events happen. We are not very aware of our flexibility surrounding this. Behavioral studies show people think their lives will not be satisfactory after suffering catastrophic injuries. However, after therapy, we seem to be able to adjust to our new lives for the most part. We even find our lives to be rewarding. That puts us as decision-makers having to judge how we currently feel about our different options and their outcomes, and how we will feel in the future if we are still experiencing such outcomes. It seems like a lot.

Chapter 6

The View from Here

From the Inside

We have shed light on the paradigm shift from IC to SDM. Sometimes we have placed ourselves within the paradigm to look at events, like the actors in a performance see events and people in the play through the script. At other times we have looked at the paradigms from the outside as if we were the audience for the play. The people participating in the paradigm have a focus and an interest in certain paradigm features. They are interested in making it better from the inside. They ask questions like, "Can we make this better by giving patients videos rather than a piece of paper describing the options?" Using and working in the paradigm presents its own struggles and puzzles. I experienced those challenges in the wild. That experience did inform me in ways the bird's-eye view does not. There are time pressures on everyone involved. The variety of capabilities in patients and health care providers makes it hard to produce a one-fits-all solution. However, one does not have to resort to a bird's-eye view to have phenomena to explore. Let us explore how we got here looking from the inside.

The IC paradigm was found wanting by the stakeholders. They eventually became aware that the activity's objectives were not being met. This was seen from within the paradigm. A pivotal articulation of this was that patient rights were not being protected. From within, you didn't really have to articulate that this was a goal of the activity. This is typical of work from within a paradigm. You see the problem through the paradigm lens, but you don't notice the lens itself. When we treated IC as a paradigm, its flaws stood out. The major puzzle was around information flow. It took many years of court decisions and attempts to plug the holes before people gave up.

The IC paradigm was about to undergo a shift. The shift was due to the information issue and how it presented an obstacle to protecting patient rights. Yet, as we have seen, it prevented patients from making good decisions. The focus of the stakeholders was twofold at the time. They were concerned with the conveyance of information but also letting go of their control. The fear was a utilitarian one. Allowing patients to make the decisions would inevitably lead to bad outcomes. There must be a better way. Shared decision-making came upon the scene. The concerns from within suggest that there are two goals in the paradigm of the encounter between the health care provider and patient.

The initial goal of the encounter is to achieve a good outcome. We really do not go to the health care provider seeking protection of our rights. We go to get better or stay well. There is an ethical restriction on the way we get there. Those restrictions involve respect for patient autonomy and self-determination. This becomes a goal or objective of the encounter as well. One can question whether we need to stick with both goals if the combination causes such problems. Let us look at the sciences and paradigm shifts there.

Science has the goals of prediction and explanation. The theories falling under the physics paradigm were fantastic at predicting. Current physics theories are the best for predicting. Do they explain the world as well as Newtonian physics? Some argued that quantum mechanics did not explain phenomena well as in the Einstein Bohr debates in the first half of the twentieth century. It depends upon what one means by "explaining." The point here is that paradigms can have more than one goal. What if a paradigm succeeds at one goal but not the other? The history of paradigm shifts can be instructive here.

The history of physics serves the point well. The goals are to predict and explain the physical world. We hope to "understand" the universe through physics. The paradigm of the seventeenth century was that physics could explain the world and predict the future. The paradigm involved the use of controlled experiments, which resulted in measurements. My favorite, but boring, example is a billiards table. The balls sit on the table, and one of the players picks up a cue. The player chalks up the tip and carefully aims at the white ball to strike another. If one observes and measures the player's stroke in terms of the angle, force, and spin imparted on the white ball, one can predict how the others will move about. The physics of it should be able to predict what will happen given all the initial conditions—the placement of all the balls on the table, their mass, the angle of the cue ball, its speed, and its spin. Given these conditions, physics equations will predict where everything will end up. It will also explain why this happens based on the laws of physics that apply to the situation. You may remember Force = Mass*Acceleration as an example. These equations explain why the balls move the way they do after striking and predict each of their paths.

It is possible that, at some point, the equations do not relate to any "model" of the universe. It is just math. The wave-particle duality of phenomena back in the early twentieth century shocked physicists. The math worked great at predicting what would happen, but it was (and is, I would argue) puzzling. *Puzzling* is not where we want to be with explanations. Maybe science need not *explain* phenomena in the sense we understand the term "explaining." I might understand the math, but I cannot relate it to my experience in any way. In any case, much history has happened since then as physicists try to understand the duality and other puzzles, even though math has not changed. The predictions are still spot-on. The explanations involve things such as pilot waves (Choudhary), all possible paths simultaneously (Feynman), and others. The drive to understand is part of the physics paradigm, as exhibited by physicists. It is a sociological phenomenon. I do not see prediction and explanation as having a logical connection, even though they are often paired and with some satisfactory results. In physics, the drive to explain what appears to be inexplicable has led to various experiments and theories that posit explanatory solutions. This is normal, and giving up on explanations as part of the scientific paradigm is not in the cards now. There is no reason to give up on it.

I think we are at the same point in our paradigm here. It is very difficult to tease out the goals of the encounter. The overall purpose of the encounter is to get the best outcome possible. There are ethical restrictions to this which involve ensuring that the process of getting there involves respect for the patient's autonomy. As someone who was a nurse, an ethics consultant in the hospital setting, and a patient, the difference between obtaining a certain physiological state and my preferences did not diverge often. My experience is that the realm of choices presented did not require a long, drawn-out process of weighing this that and the other thing. Luckily, most of my infirmities have been acute rather than chronic. The alternative courses of treatment were not significantly different in efficacy or adverse effects. Most of the time, these are Fast and Frugal types of interactions. I would contend rightfully so. What most patients and I appreciate is the respect that my physicians pay to bring me into the decision-making process. I feel like I own the decision. I am more compliant with the therapy (Kaplan).

As we have seen, the goals intertwine. The best outcome needs to be defined through patient values, which might go beyond physiological states. This helps to drive the interaction. The goals of the interaction cannot be accomplished without sharing this information. These insights extend back into the philosophical literature.

This work has put some meat on these old bones but shows that this sharing has to happen to meet the goals of the paradigm.

Historically, most work about paradigms is performed from within the paradigm. Those most familiar with engaging the paradigm know when something is off base. These stakeholders prioritize what they think is important in conducting the work. This is the current situation from within.

A review of the published articles yields an idea of where efforts are being expended. Categorizing the research is a bit challenging. Nevertheless, here we go. Efforts by the stakeholders have involved studying ways to make the information from the medical side more digestible. This began prior to the shift to SDM. Second, there is research into measuring the outcomes of the encounter. Third, there is research into how best to recognize a successful SDM encounter.

As for patient comprehension, there have been and continue to be studies performed about patient comprehension. One systematic review article by Glaser focuses on various interventions to improve patient comprehension. The findings are interesting in many ways. We can improve over just handing over the standard consent forms. We can offer written information at the second grade reading level. Other mixed modalities, such as audio-visual, interactive digital, and verbal discussion with test feedback, show improvements.

The studies did not include an understanding of the patient's own preferences. We know how important that must be, especially for SDM. This is not to say that research into value clarification is not taking place (Witteman 801-820). The studies falling under the review look at successful interventions as reducing regret or uncertainty of choosing among competing values. Some studies look at the relationship between the interventions and how they affect the congruence of the decision with the patient's stated value.

It would be like telling you I like chocolate a lot more than vanilla and then choosing a vanilla cone. This would come under the category of an intervention needed to make the information more digestible. The difference is that the information is coming from the patient.

Another category is the testing of the outcomes. Researchers have noted that communication with patients and patient comprehension have been assessed (Pietrzykowski). There has been a follow-up of health outcomes (Greenfield et al., 1985; Kaplan et al., 1989). Looking at a more recent article, poor use of SDM resulted in all kinds of poor outcomes (Hughes et al., 2018). These results do not cut across all therapeutic areas. More research would be needed to validate the claims of SDM promoting positive outcomes. It should be noted that the outcomes in question are patient-reported outcomes, although in one case, health resource utilization is used as a proxy (Hughes). The health resource in question was emergency department visits. Patients who participated in a good SDM scenario showed up in the emergency department less frequently than those who did not. Poor SDM was also associated with poor physical and mental health as self-reports from the patients.

These are fortunate findings. One of the questions we have going into the success of the paradigm is defining the success of its use in achieving the goals. One of these goals is successful outcomes. Of course, we know that the outcomes can be termed a success from both a physiological view and a patient values perspective. The study by Hughes uses patient self-reports about how they feel post-intervention. These studies tend to measure patient satisfaction with the process and/or the results. We have shown that the process's success may not lead to a desirable outcome. We also know all too well from behavioral economic studies that hindsight is not 20/20. Was a good result due to our makeup, experience, and information, or were we just lucky or unlucky if the results were not what we wanted?

The current situation is that much work needs to be done on evaluating outcome measures for SDM. There are some components that the researchers agree upon in large part. Besides the measure fulfilling reliability and validity standards of scales, they should measure patient satisfaction with the process, patient regret after the intervention, and patient dissonance from their values. There is also a lot of research on health care provider behavior. When I searched on PubMed in Feb 2023, I found over 3700 articles published in the past five years on the subject of shared decision-making. PubMed is a database concerned with medicine.

We can draw a few broad conclusions from the studies in decision-making. There is a lot of activity. It stretches across many of the necessary components of executing a successful SDM encounter (Benson, 2016). There are some 175 biases which he organized into 20 strategies. To quote William James (331 out of 520), it is a bit of a "blooming buzzing confusion." The next move by Benson is quite clever. He organized and grouped the strategies according to what problems were being addressed. He produced four types of strategies: Too much information, not enough meaning, need to act fast, and what to remember. These are Fast and Frugal types of strategies. Unfortunately, these strategies can be quite flawed in the wild. I emphasize the "can" here, as they do not have to be flawed. Circumstances make a difference.

Given the scope of these findings, it is interesting to note that within the decision sciences, there is debate on the findings of these research studies. Apparently, they are awfully hard to replicate (Open Science Collaboration). This presents quite a conundrum. Replication of an experiment is important to ascertain the believability of the results. It doesn't mean that the original study was wrong, but it does throw it into doubt.

Sometimes we see opposite effects, like when framing scenarios positively or negatively. In some contexts, we choose to go for the positively framed choice and sometimes the negative one. A good general rule about how to frame options for patients remains hidden.

Given the substantial number of biases in the literature and a rather big question about their significance, it is hard to see how to proceed. A very good and interesting book by Blumenthal-Barty tackles these issues. The work comes at the issues by seeing where autonomy can be protected, but the more pernicious biases are reduced. These are just the practical measures that SDM needs. These measures should not undermine autonomy but support the decision-making process. Does this take away patient autonomy?

That is an interesting question. I don't think being self-determined or autonomous means that you cannot have help. There are restrictions on how and when to give such assistance. Discussions on these topics go beyond the scope of the work here. After all, we are interested in paradigms and their shifts. SDM has its two goals; if research shows that they cannot be met, then something must give.

Behavioral Economics research gives us all pause about considering ourselves competent decision-makers. There are so many land mines in our way that it is a wonder we last as long as we do. However, on an ethical note, patients do no worse than health care providers in this regard. Once we see that competency is a relative term, then the goal changes from wresting away control of the decision to supporting it.

There is a lot left to do. Much of the basic research does not meet acceptable standards for conclusions. Typically, 50 percent seems to be the mark. The good news is that from the "here" of the inside, there have not been insurmountable barriers. We can project that there will be arguments about what is "rational," "competent," a "preference," "autonomous" and so on. It is the nature of the beast. What will succeed will be where the researchers take us. They may find adequate ways of dealing with biases or our heuristic ways of thinking. Or they may decide it isn't a workable paradigm. That decision could be based on the right reasons (the paradigm cannot accommodate the facts) or incorrectly, such as believing that the paradigm must be right even if contradicts the facts. One such mistake would be to think that patients are not competent because of a one-time failure. The area where I see this needing to be worked out is with decisions that seem to fly in the face of the patient's statements about what they value. Let us look at a scenario.

A patient states on a values clarification form that they prefer maintaining their appearance over increasing the likelihood of increased longevity. I had such a patient during my nursing internship at the VA. He had tongue cancer, but it was not visible to the public. Every day he would stand in front of the bathroom mirror and comb his hair meticulously. In fact, he dressed meticulously while in the hospital. Even though he had said looking good was the most important thing to him, even more important than increased lifespan, he elected to have the surgery. Something doesn't add up.

The options include the possibility that actions speak louder than words. I mean, who hasn't thought they valued something more until faced with the situation? Another possibility is that the patient is letting circumstances get in the way of their thinking process. They get so afraid that they just opt for what they think others want. They don't realize that they are caught in a contradiction. They aren't thinking "clearly." We will say a bit more about this issue, but first, let us clear up whether this makes them incompetent.

I think my version of competency accommodates this type of real-world scenario. The ladder example handles one interpretation of this patient's surgery. Assuming that appearance is his ultimate goal, he is not making the best choice here. He is unable to exercise it because of the fear of dying. Even so, he remains competent under my analysis. We need to respect the decision. Those who have recommended a nudge to prevent this error have not suggested taking the decision away from the patient.

How we value and create preferences and what we want is challenging for us. I mean, I want to eat foods that I know are not good for my health or longevity. I value my health and longevity. I want those things as well. When I am under stress, I want to eat more now than live somewhat longer. My decision is not well thought out. Immediate gratification is preferred to a delayed one. If you ask me what I want, more longevity or this piece of chocolate, I would probably state that I would want to live longer. If confronted with an actual candy bar, I clearly have been opting for the chocolate. Maybe I really want both, but I can only have one. As the people trying to get the patient to make the call, it is difficult. I think we are a long way from understanding preferences, desires, and values, although we often use them interchangeably. Now the best I can see is to point out what the patient said before to ensure they understand the discordance. Would they give you the same ordering when confronted with this seeming contradiction? More research needs to be done.

My view from the inside is that the research needs to be reliable. Much, if not most, stems from behavioral economics, and until reliability can be established, we should not jump the gun. It tells me more about running the experiments than the results about how people think. My guess is that much of it will turn out to be valuable information, and some coarse generalizations are true. For instance, framing has an effect. Exactly how needs to be put in the framework of a hypothesis that can be confirmed or disconfirmed by an experiment. Many of the articles and books I have read fall into the category of excellent hypothesis generators, but the results are not true for everybody. Take the famous disease study. The scenarios are to frame an intervention as saving lives or not, and either with certainty or probability. An important feature of the results is that most of us respond to this effect similarly, somewhere around 70 percent. Of course, that means that 30 percent do not. The results are probable themselves about how we choose. There is a cautionary tale here about our worries. Let us move back from all of this and take a bird's-eye view.

From the Outside

I have had the experience of being inside the world of the encounter as a nurse, ethics consultant, and clinical researcher. In addition, I have spent many hours outside the paradigm as a philosopher. The vantage point of looking in has allowed me to see how the various elements work or don't work together. It has allowed me to shift my own perspective. Treating the activity of the encounter as having a paradigm conjures up its own connections. It must have a goal for the activity. The participants share at least some rudimentary understanding and expectations of what will happen. This perspective yields other areas that are not entirely evident when studying the trees. We know that decision-making capacity plays a role, including the ability to comprehend information and much more. It is intimately related to the right to make the decision and self-determination. It is also related to making good choices. Things are lined up well so long as we can successfully define competence and decision-making. I think we have done so. This begins the journey toward understanding rationality in this practical context. We have taken some pains to get this on the right footing. It isn't deductive reasoning, nor is it gambling. It falls between and lines up better with either Fast and Frugal approaches or a more cursory Bentham calculus.

When we take a step back, there are some things to note. Paradigm shifts have historically happened from within the discipline among the actual stakeholders. Scientists trying to solve their puzzles come up with a new paradigm. They decidedly have not relied on the philosophical community for input. This doesn't mean some other perspective cannot be incorporated. That would take a logical argument. Whether it will or will not take in these other considerations is a matter of empirical conjecture. I hope that, in this case, the researchers are more open to understanding what they are assuming from within the paradigm so they can move more quickly in establishing or moving on from SDM. Here is a brief review.

Researchers should be aware of the philosophical debates about rationality, preferences, autonomy, and derivatives. Understanding how these impact the paradigm could lead to quicker results about keeping certain items or abandoning them. Here are a few of the many philosophers that have engaged on these topics. I have limited the citations to two here. Some researchers do this now (Blumenthal-Barty, 2021). Others have written about topics apart from BE. Philosophers have discussed rationality in great detail (Parfit, 1981; Audi, 2001). Preferences and values play a role, as we have seen. The philosophers range deep into our past with Bentham. More modern philosophers have published on axiology—the study of value (Rescher, 2005; Findlay, 1970). Autonomy and freedom have a longstanding place in philosophy (Kant, 1785; Audi, 2001). The bibliography contains additional authors.

The questions I find most relevant, and this is based on my private opinions/interests, are the following:

1. Is connecting autonomy to rationality necessary?
2. Does distinguishing wanting something from goals holds up?
3. How do we conceptually look at a success rate for these types of decisions?
4. How should I handle my future self, given my poor predicting power?
5. Should we just give our preferences to Artificial Intelligence, and would that satisfy the requirements of self-determination?

Let's turn briefly to each.

1. We understand that Kant made a strong case for the intricate relationship between autonomy and rationality. I suspected this was part of his larger program that separated the empirical sciences from ethics and religion. In large measure, the mechanistic interpretations of science via Newton's laws would make ethical choices a sham. It does seem we believe that moral choices need to be made freely, and Newton's determinism blocks that approach. Getting the concept of rationality right is a bit of a bear. Kant's version is not so much about prudent decisions as it is about ethical ones. The conceptual analyses around autonomy involve some parsing from liberty. Liberty is typically cast as free from outside coercive influences. What is interesting to me here is that we could consider autonomy to be more a matter of following your preferences without referencing who figures it out. I think that would be different from our current understanding of the paradigm. I liken it a bit to the tale of Ulysses having his sailors tie him to the mast of the ship so he can hear the Sirens, but his men cannot hear his orders. His orders prior to that

sail will stand: the ship must not crash into the rocks. Anything else between here and past the rocks is to be ignored. Just get me there.

There is a feeling I have that this is not fulfilling. It may be more psychological than conceptual. The more I participate in the decision, the more control I feel I have. My clinical experience is that most patients feel this way. It is important to give patients real choices in the hospital setting and treat them as active participants and not as passive receptacles of care. They don't feel so much at the mercy of others. In the sense that we get to pick the alternative, we are the masters of our fate. If the information about the prognosis and the alternatives is accurate, then making the selection seems powerful. The "I" gets to make a choice, not the "you." No one else is determining my fate. What could go wrong, though, is my making a bad choice given my values. But does that mean I am not determining my fate? At this point, I think not. It would explain why I feel I screwed up if I made misjudgments while thinking it through and have regret. It also leaves someone self-determined and autonomous when they hand over the decision-making to someone else. This is certainly worthy of consideration. If I were still a graduate philosophy student, this would be greater than a one-pint discussion.

2. Another troubling component is the wants v. goals. It might be the same as the immediate v. delayed gratification issue. However, I think there is more to this. The models about goals and the discussions in the literature have a view of a well-ordered preference ranking. I am, quite frankly, jealous. My immediate preferences are known to me, but they are not that well-ordered. What I say and what I do diverge significantly in some areas. As Walt Whitman wrote: "Do I contradict myself? Very well, then I contradict myself. I am large, I contain multitudes" (Whitman, *Songs of Myself* 51). I want or have as goals multiple states, which I cannot possess as a matter of practicality. All the rational reflection may be without merit for values clarification. This doesn't preclude a clarifying response as to

why my feelings are misleading on this point. If patients flip-flop all of the time, then how should one proceed? Is the purpose of sharing information to get buy in and compliance of the patient, and the current view of self-determination to achieve a goal is a useful myth?

3. The success rate is relative to the task at hand and how others perform. Success is about processes or outcomes. This really has to be answered. Consider the following scenarios:

    a. Some patients state that their bodily integrity is more important than longevity. Of these, a portion of patients chose not to have surgery. They died early as a result. The patients say they are happy with their choice any way prior to expiring. Was this a successful decision? Does happiness indicate success?

    b. Suppose some other patients make the same choice with the same stated goals. Unfortunately, these patients are now regretting their former choice. Was this a successful decision? Does regret indicate failure?

    c. Some other patients decide to have the surgery even though it goes against their stated goals. They want to live longer. They do live longer. Was this a successful decision?

    d. Some patients decide to have surgery and regret it even though they live longer. Was this a successful decision? Again, does regret play a role?

The question for these is, how can we measure the success of the decision? Is it that it conforms to a standard of processing? Or is it solely results based? The answers to that question should play a role in how concerned we should be about the process. If the only thing that matters at the end of the day is the patient's perception of having navigated to good results based on their future state, then let's nudge.

4. The examples in (3) play a role in future self-issues. All along, we have been making assumptions about the self who makes evaluations about goals. Even in my thesis in 1984, I recognized there was a problem of which self gets to make the evaluation. My current and near-term versions of myself will certainly have to bear sacrifices and/or benefits from my decisions. Of course, they can reach out to a far more distant self and project how that distant self will feel tenuous at best. In that work, I explored social welfare economics as an approach to giving each version of my "self" equal weight in the decision. To be frank, I couldn't think of another approach that made much sense. There are all sorts of problems with that approach as well. You run into Arrow's Impossibility Theorem (Arrow,) and it remains a mystery to me how to treat these variations in the self. Needless to say, philosophers have been contending with the continuity of the self anyway (Hume; Kant; Parfit). The issues of regret have a more modern treatment, as in Sour Grapes (Sen pp219-238). Elster also deals with future directives, and the example of Ulysses comes from his excellent work.

5. The last item of most interest is AI. It is good at absorbing enormous amounts of data and calculating from there. A question that comes from this is if a patient puts in a preference, can the rational process be performed more reliably by AI? Suppose the answer is yes. It doesn't feel as paternalistic to me if I affirm using the computer to calculate my choice. But I think that is outside the SDM paradigm. The value of SDM is the communication that should be taking place. Laying out the alternatives is not simple because they involve pathways to the end results. The paths need to be discussed. Patients need to imagine life under each alternative. Some of the difficult situations, as in 3c, demonstrate a lack of value congruence. I do not find it odd that we chose things at odds with what we stated we would choose. As a practical matter in important medical decisions, we would want to remind the patients that they said something different.

They could have changed their minds to what they originally said. Alternatively, they could say they were hasty in their original statement. They could also say that they can't decide. They do not know what they want. It is a problem. The use of AI may end up stifling further discussion to clarify choices, or it could be used as a tool for the patient self-reflection, if that is the path they are willing to risk.

My closing thoughts are that the SDM paradigm is still in its early stages. Many people are excited and motivated enough to perform research during its infancy. The researchers are suffering the pangs of new realms of research, such as BE, but are making great progress. SDM appears to be getting more of a coherent paradigm as theories of understanding, projection, and medical ethics feed into each other. The number of published articles in peer review journals is outstanding.

As a former practitioner at the bedside, I have to say the communication process and respect for patients have been a long transition. It has challenges for those on the provider side of which those outside the field are most likely unaware. Long shifts, too little time, and numerous non-care demands put people under pressure. Time is an ally long sought to make for more successful interactions. Costs and staffing play against that. Any tools and research that reduce the burdens associated with the encounter are welcome.

As a former bioethics consultant at the bedside, I can truthfully say that communication was the most frequent issue. People say stuff to each other all the time. Often, they are talking about one thing in order to not talk about something else. They are making decisions quickly and without a tremendous amount of thought because the cost of going through the process is too burdensome under the circumstances. I have always believed that we shouldn't let perfect get in the way of the good. We can help patients, but if the expectation is that the decisions will be perfect, then I expect us to be terribly disappointed. Remember, our definition of competency was being good enough, if you will.

What I believe is happening with the advent of SDM is that we are helping patients go through the decision process, even if it is flawed. Patients are showing an appreciation for the effort. They are more compliant with their therapies since they are "owning" their therapies. The more we can help everyone, the better off we are. The more we approach the process as a team working together, the less we will feel burdened. The research from all areas is worthwhile, even the ones that close down certain avenues that were going to be dead ends.

Appendix A

A Philosophical Analysis of Competency

It is time to give an example of putting significant detail into the SDM paradigm. The place of competency is pivotal in many ways to the paradigm. It has at least two directions in which it travels through the paradigm. As in the Schloendorff case, it earmarks a patient with the right to make the choice. At the same time, it provides for more successful decisions. The concept relies on the concept of "can". In its most basic form, if you are competent at something, we could say you can do it. In Chapter 5, we introduced the fact that "can" has various meanings. The way in which the meaning of "can" is most appropriately used in this context is of vital importance. I have argued that it is related to the concept of success. In addition, the success rate is relative to the human performance of the task. It leaves the "can" of opportunity and abilities as being relevant. Here we are going to push through various options for defining having the ability to provide more meat on the bones.

A few explanatory notes for the foregoing are in order. The analysis and definitions attempt to clarify the concept of competency while referring to the ladder-climbing example in the text. The "P" in (P1) and so on are the propositions being presented. "S" is the subject performing the actions. "A" is the action. If and only if (iff) is used to express a logical condition.

One illustration of this logical condition can be directly borrowed from Plato. The definition of knowledge is that it is a justified true belief. Using our abstract formulation, it would become "S knows that P iff S believes P is true and S is justified in believing P is true and P is true. The item to the left of the 'iff' is true only when all the items to the right are true. Or if you prefer

143

right to left, whenever all the items to the right are true, then the item to the left of the 'iff' is also true. It might look like T 'iff' T is always true."

This is a typical set of philosophical attempts. We propose a definition of competency and then find counterexamples. This leads us to redefine competency to meet the objections. This is not unlike the court's struggles when dealing with informed consent. Let the games begin. The first go looks like this:

(Pl): S is competent to do A iff S has the ability to do A and S has all the abilities to exercise the ability to do A.

(Pl) satisfies the intuitions concerning competency in the examples presented thus far. For example, the ladder climber has the physical ability to make it up each individual rung. The climber has the opportunity. What S lacks is the ability to overcome a fear. Without this ability, which is an ability this person needs to exercise the climbing ability, the person is not competent to climb up to the top of the ladder. A medical example might seem more pertinent.

Suppose a medical student is particularly gifted with his/her/their hands. They/he/she intends to go into surgical practice. Practice on cadavers indicates that this student will be a great surgeon. Nevertheless, after repeated attempts at working on living humans, this student has tremors that make successful surgery impossible. This student is not a competent surgeon.

Now suppose that the chief surgeon fools the student by slipping in a live patient who has been made hypothermic. The student does not tremble, believing that the body is a cadaver. The student does well, being able to exercise the appropriate surgical abilities. Yet, I don't think we would consider the student a competent surgeon. The student can exercise the ability without having the ability to exercise the surgical ability.

(Pl) appears to account for the previously cited intuitions concerning competency. Take the example of an obviously competent patient who is given no information concerning treatments or prognosis. Withholding this information deprives the patient of the opportunity of making a truly competent decision. Yet, the patient is not incompetent. A lack of opportunity does not imply incompetency. (Pl) does not entail that the person has to have the opportunity to do A to be competent and therefore is in accordance with this example.

(Pl) does entail that the person must have the ability to do A to be competent. Surely that must be the most basic requirement for the concept of competency.

(Pl) also accounts for our intuitions concerning the ladder case.

(Pl) appears to handle a variety of intuitions concerning competency. Still, to this point, the analysis needs more detail to provide any guidelines for determining when someone is competent. The reason is that the concept of ability is central to the definition, but that concept has yet to be analyzed.

There are two analyses of the concept of the ability which appear in the literature and seem most appropriate for our purposes. Although they differ in some details, they share one common feature: they make the concept of success part of the meaning of the concept of ability.

Kaufman proposes the following as an analysis of the meaning of ability: "'the person has the ability to do A' means 'the person is in a certain condition C (C being the appropriate state of the organism brought to a certain pitch of development), such that, given an opportunity, C causes the person to succeed in A'ing an appropriate percentage of the time (where the unspecified complexity of C determines the appropriate percentage) if he should try A'"(Kaufman, 1970). I will call this definition (P2).

(P2) has a variety of important features. Of particular interest is the success feature. In (P2), there is a certain level of success that is necessary for there to be an ability. Suppose the person succeeds an appropriate percentage of the time, and that success is due to the person's condition (rather than some "external" circumstance). In that case, the person has the ability to do A.

D. Locke offers a similar proposal. "The person has the ability to do A, so long as the person's constitution and history are such that given the opportunity and the motivation, the person himself, by his actions, will standardly bring it about that the person does A" (Hereafter (P2')). (Locke, 1973-1974)

(P2'), I think should be considered as a "success-type" definition. What else could the "standardly bring it about that the person does A" mean? The standard in each case would need to be explored, but the concept of success would still be employed.

There is an apparent problem with this type of analysis. M. Brand has proposed a counterexample to any analysis, including the concept of success as part of the meaning of ability. His example involves a perfectly able golfer for whom miraculous wind gusts interfere with his ability to sink short putts. The wind universally gets in his way no matter when and where he putts it. This golfer is never successful. By definition, he has the ability to sink short putts if it were not for those nasty gusts of wind, which are miraculous. As Brand concludes, "Being in the most appropriate state under the most favorable conditions is compatible with never successfully exercising one's ability" (Brand, 1970).

Of course, this counterexample purportedly gives us an instance of someone who has an ability but is unsuccessful in exercising it. The two analyses ((P2) and (P2')) require some success and, therefore, cannot account for that ability. So, given that the golfer has the ability and is unsuccessful, we would have a true counterexample. There are some problems with this interpretation of the counterexample, which is that he has the ability but is unsuccessful. At least some of these problems can be attributed to how the golfer's action is described. Which events in the sequence are to be attributed to the golfer and which are not? These break down naturally into two categories. Either the golfer's action is present until and just through the stroking of the ball, or the action includes rolling the ball until it comes to rest. Either sequence could legitimately be called putting.

Let us take the former description first. Here, the golfer ends after contact has been made with the ball. After that, the consequences are beyond the golfer's control. The environment will take over. An able golfer usually knows what the environment is like and will consider such things as wind, speed of the green, any breaks in the green, etc. when stroking the ball.

If we look at the golfer's action this way, we find that his action in the counterexample is analogous to throwing a pair of dice. This is because the gusts of wind are, by definition, miraculous and cannot, as a result, be considered. Likewise, when we try to roll a seven, we throw the dice and, because of an environment we cannot take into account, they may turn up seven. That we cannot consider these factors when we roll the dice shows that we do not have the ability to roll a seven. It is a matter of luck. Sinking putts in miraculous gusts of wind would also be due to luck, and there is no reason to suppose that anyone could possess the ability to sink putts under those circumstances.

To clarify this point, suppose we lived on a planet where golfers and golf courses were all subjected to miraculous wind gusts. Of course, no one can sink putts here with any regularity because of the wind. There is little, if any, the temptation to think that anyone has the ability to sink putts under these circumstances.

The result of the fictional planet example eliminates the force of the counterexample, for there is no reason to suppose, as the counterexample does, that our golfer has the ability to sink putts in miraculous gusts of wind.

The fact is that the counterexample gains its force because the golfer does stroke the ball correctly so that it would sink if there were no miraculous gusts of wind. Why else would it be supposed that the golfer had the ability to sink putts? But this maneuver reintroduces the concept of success back into the analysis. Success would be necessary for some hypothetical standard situations where the conditions are within certain limits. If those conditions existed, the golfer would be successful a certain percentage of the time.

The other way of describing the action itself is to include the events which occur after the ball has been stroked. Therefore, the golfer's action is sinking putts, not just stroking the ball. Part of what this means is that there are basic standard conditions (vague as they may be) that are part of the act of sinking putts. This is what makes it the act of sinking putts and not something else. Miraculous gusts of wind make this act different than we normally think of when we consider sinking putts.

Applying the preceding results to the counterexample, we find that although the golfer is the only one plagued with the miraculous gusts of wind, this changes the nature of the act about to be performed. This golfer is not attempting to sink putts (which is one act) but is attempting to sink miraculous putts (which is a different act). This different act depends upon luck for success, not ability. Our golfer does not have the ability to sink miraculous putts, and the lack of success shows this. Yet, the golfer, by hypothesis, does have the ability to sink putts. This fact turns out to be irrelevant under this description of the act.

The upshot of all of this is that Brand is both right and wrong when he states that success is not part of the meaning of ability. He is right if actual success is meant to be part of the meaning of ability. His example shows that clearly. However, his example does not speak directly to the issue of whether the concept of success plays an essential role in the meaning of ability. If anything, the above analysis indicates that a level of success in the hypothetical standard situation is a necessary condition for there to be an ability.

Up to now, the analysis has been negative in nature. Brand's counterexample has been shown to be ineffective against a success-type analysis, yet this alone does not show that the concept of success is part of the meaning of ability; the question remains as to whether there are any reasons for including the concept of success in the analysis.

To answer this question, I will employ the following strategy: I will argue that there are good reasons for thinking that the concept of success is part of the meaning of the concept of ability. If it is, then it can be shown that it (the concept of success) is part of the epistemology of ability,

I will also deal with the alternative position that the concept of success is not part of the meaning of the concept of ability. The arguments for this position will be presented. These arguments, however, will also imply that the concept of success is part of the epistemology of ability. So even if it (the concept of success) is not part of the meaning of the concept of an ability, it is how we verify that an ability is present.

The concept of success plays a role that is essential in the epistemological analysis of ability, regardless of whether it is part of the meaning of that term. I think it is embedded in the idea of having the ability, but even if I am incorrect, it clearly is related.

What we will do is provide good reasons for thinking that the concept of success is involved in the meaning of ability. The linkage between the concepts results from the fact that when people have an ability, it is always an ability to do something. The ability is linked to an action of some sort. There is always a performance in mind when someone thinks of a specific ability. If one were to describe a specific ability, one would describe an act. The description of the act is a description of a successful outcome.

The ability to hit a forehand in tennis will serve as a suitable example. One receives the ball on the racket-hand side of the body, draws the racket back toward the baseline, and brings it forward, hitting the ball with the face of the racket, sending it over the net and into the opponent's court. The ability was just described in terms of a successful performance. Of course, for it to be an ability would necessitate doing it several times, which means several successes. Hence, success does play a role in explicating the concept of ability.

A different and opposing point of view would be that the concept of success does not form part of the meaning of the concept of ability. The ability and the act are separate items, not connected analytically. The description of the ability does not include the description of the act. The ability is something the agent possesses, whereas the act is not.

To illustrate this, the ability to leap will serve as an example. The ability to leap can be described according to the physiological characteristics of the agent. The muscles will have fibers of a certain number and length. Nerves will be innervating various muscles in appropriate ways, when synapsed they will cause a successful leap (again under the appropriate conditions), but the leap itself is an act of the agent, not part of the agent's constitution; there is a difference between the constitution of the agent and the acts which that constitution can cause.

The point here is that the concept of success is tied to the act. A description of a successful leap, according to this view, would only include the description of the act; it would not include a description of the constitution of the agent. Yet it is the constitution of the agent that is the ability. Therefore, success would not be analytically tied to the concept of ability.

Granting that there is this conceptual wedge, does that preclude the concept of success in the epistemological analysis? The answer is no. No, because how we would come to know that the person's constitution could cause A to occur is to notice that A occurs when the person employs that constitution (under the appropriate circumstance). A certain level of success is the evidence we would use to decide that that constitution was indeed the ability necessary to cause A to occur. If A failed to occur, we would reconsider whether this constitution was an ability. Once again, successful outcomes will be the essential evidence for determining whether someone has an ability (*ceteris paribus*). The concept of success is part of the epistemology of ability under this alternative too.

At this point, I would like to present an analysis that considers the preceding discussion. This analysis also deals with Brand's counterexample effectively by employing the concept of success in a hypothetical way, thus removing the force of his counterexample.

(P2") the person has the ability to do A if and only if the person's constitution and history are such that if the person were to attempt to do a significant number of times in a hypothetical (possible) world where the standard conditions for A'ing obtain, then the person would succeed in doing A an appropriate percentage of the time.

This analysis does meet the objections presented by the Brand counterexample. Yet there is a counterexample to (P2"). Suppose that there is another golfer who is a real klutz. In fact, to call him a golfer is to insult others who have taken up the sport. The klutz, by hypothesis, does not have the ability to sink putts. Even though conditions are perfect, our klutz would not normally succeed. Suppose that the conditions are perfect. Suppose, further, that our klutz is so klutzy that as the club face approaches the ball (at the wrong angle, of course), he slips, falls, and hits it inadvertently but perfectly. The ball rolls in. Each time the klutz goes to hit the ball, another mishap occurs. An unintentional but nonetheless perfect stroke occurs. Success occurs, the conditions are perfect, and the stroke is due to the klutz's constitution and history. Yet the klutz, by hypothesis, does not have the ability even though he satisfies the conditions outlined in (P2"). The problem is that the person's actions, which bring about the perfect stroke, are not intentional. To correct this, I offer the following:

(P2*): the person has the ability to do A if and only if the person's constitution and history are such that if the person were to attempt A in a possible world where the standard conditions for A'ing obtain, then the person, by the person's own intentional actions caused by the person's constitution and history, would succeed in doing A an appropriate percentage of the time.

(P2*) meets head-on the problem posed by the klutz example by including the intentional aspect of the person's actions. It also distinguishes luck from the ability, as the success of the action is due to the person's constitution and history and not some external circumstance. It also considers the concept of success.

(P2*) serves as the framework from which the epistemological inquiry will take place. It indicates the questions that will have to be answered to know if the person has the ability to do A. These questions include, but are not limited to, the following:

What is the nature of the act to be performed?

What are the standard conditions for the performance of this act?

What is the acceptable percentage of success necessary to grant that the person has the ability to do A? Sports, as in other endeavors, are set by norms of how other people perform. In baseball, getting a hit 25 percent of the time or more makes you a successful major-league hitter if that percentage is from a big-league competition. Golf already has its norms called par. We are not so precise with decision-making under uncertainty. We can say that the definition offered here means we need to consider the standard conditions for making successful decisions and try to make those happen in the HCP-patient interaction.

We should conclude from the above that the success rates of decisions are critical to the paradigm of SDM. It also means that a person needs an opportunity to exercise the ability to make decisions. Any possible support the health care team can give patients is critical to success.

Appendix B

Challenges to Utility Comparisons – Cardinality

We have noted in the text that the expected value model or any utility model relying on the equations requires the ability to compare these values across different dimensions. This is linked to the decision-maker's consistency and ability to compare across dimensions. We note that one of the most seductive pieces of the EV model is its seeming objectivity. We're going to come up with a decision case that looks cardinal and is cardinal, but the numbers are still somewhat arbitrary.

First, let us relate this to the future vs. present self issue. In 1960 Kenneth Arrow pointed out some logical difficulties with the conditions in the context of combining votes from three or more voters into a winner. This problem only applies if the same self (meaning the same set of preferences) exists with different preference orderings over time. He discovered an actual paradox in what are excellent rules for making decisions. Here we are only dealing with one person, but the assumption is that the person has the same set of preferences over time. If not, they will have past, current, and future selves. It is unclear if that makes the case completely analogous to the one Arrow presented, but it is in some relevant ways. If the decision-making context for an individual is analogous in the right ways to Arrow, then we are faced with the same paradox. A paradox is not a good thing to face. In the case of an individual, there would be the self at present and other selves at different future times. The different selves would occur each time there is a change in the preference order for that self. Many selves could be voting on what constitutes a good outcome.

How does this processing model work when we are confronted with this choice issue? What can be gained by Arrow's interpersonal comparisons (those between people) for intrapersonal comparisons are those between my different selves over time.

The problem of inter-utility comparisons has usually been relegated to the world of interpersonal comparisons. Often, it has been thought that making such comparisons involved the problem of other minds. Intra-utility comparisons can happen within one individual.

Making these comparisons between people has a long history in welfare economics. MacKay has argued extensively that social welfare decision-making should have no cardinality assumptions. Cardinality means that intensities are involved, not just the order. An example is the height ordering of a class of ten children. You can compare them to one another and figure out who is the tallest and, subsequently, all the way down to who is the shortest. You do not have to resort to actual values in inches or centimeters. This would be an ordinal ranking. If you bothered to measure their heights, the tallest is 5 foot 7 inches, all the way down to the shortest, 4 foot 8 inches. This latter approach would be a cardinal ranking.

MacKay first suggested the athletic example of a polyathalon. Table 2 gives some of the correspondence between making decisions and the events.

Table 2 Comparison of Decision-Making with a Polyathalon

Decision Making over time	Polyathalon
Different Utility Functions	Different Events
Alternatives	Competitors
Preference order	Order of finish
Cardinal preference scale	Performance in time or distance

Several athletes are competing in a polyathalon event. The goal is to devise a scoring system to decide who will be the best all-around athlete. This scoring system should be rational. The International Association of Athletics (IAAF), now known as World Athletics, is the organization that puts forth the scoring system. Table 2 is part of one line from the scale of points given for different events. For example, 1000 points could be made by running 10.395 sec for the 100 m dash, or 46.17 seconds for the 400 m run, and so on.

Table 3 Partial IAAF Scoring Table for Decathlon (Barrow)

Event	1,000 pts	900 pts
100m	10.395	10.827
Long Jump	7.76	7.36
Shot Put	18.4	16.79
High Jump	2.20	2.10
400m	46.17	48.19
110m Hurdles	13.8	14.59
Discus Throw	56.17	51.4
Pole Vault	5.28	4.96
Javelin Throw	77.19	70.67
1500m	3:53.79	4:07.42

The manner in which the IAAF constructs these tables is through a formula.

The track events use the formula P=a*(b-T) **c where T is in seconds

The jumps utilize the formula P= a*(m-b) **cm where M is in cm

Throws utilize the formula P = a*(D-b) **c where D is in meters.

Each formula sets itself out as a utility function. The constants differ for different events. The different constants and formulas have some basis in actual performances and physiology. The key point here is not following the rather complex math but the fact that there is some sound way to construct these tables for establishing points. The analog to our situation is that the formulas for each event represent different utility functions. There is actually quite a literature behind the polyathalon calculations. They stem from being about physiology and the velocity or kinetic energy that a body needs to be able to impart for the particular event. Who knew? There are arguments against using physiology as the basis of points. One can argue that it should be based on the world records of the event. The use of math is seductive and gives an air of objectivity. Certainly, it is not biased in the sense of having an athlete you want to win be the winner. There are built-in biases in the assumptions. The table above will favor certain types of athletes as the current system does. The shorter sprints have more weight in scoring points.

Basically, there is an attempt to normalize the utility functions based on some standard. But it does depend upon the constants and the events. Can we do the same for utility functions? Referring to Table 3, let us see what parallels can be drawn. Each event is a different utility function, and it would be no problem assigning a maximum utility, say 1200 points. After all, why should we show a bias toward a particular utility function?

The next step is to take the results of the previous competitors in the event. This part is less clear when it comes to utility functions. One possibility is that one compares how this particular utility function has worked with this set of alternatives in the past for the individual, which is how successful it has been in satisfying the individual in the past. One would get a range or average. Unfortunately, many utility functions have to be evaluated that the individual has never possessed. This method is not available to the individual patient directly. However, it does seem possible for a person to see how well it has worked for other people with similar tastes. Here is another possible area of research for SDM. We have seen that people can be more flexible than we thought. Pointing this out to a patient making a decision gives them more information to rely on.

Even though this is possible, it generates further challenges. Treating all our possible utility functions as equals can lead to strange results. Bricker has pointed out that when one allows each utility function to be judged internally for its success and the functions are treated as equals, then counterexamples can be produced. "A can take a pill that can have two effects. First, it would cause him to become the willing slave of a wicked master: A would never again have the opportunity to exercise his free will. …And secondly, the pill would give A bias toward the actual: it would cause him always to prefer the actual to the possible, always to prefer what does happen (in his life as a slave) to what could have happened (had he never taken the pill)" (Bricker 394).

According to A's current utility function, prior to taking the pill, he would not want to become a slave. Therefore, his current utility function points to him not taking the pill. But once he has taken the pill, he will always be satisfied. The utility function of taking the pill will always yield better internal results than A's current utility function since the current function will sometimes not get satisfied. In one case, we would be a pig totally satisfied, but in the other, we might be a Socrates satisfied most of the time. Through this procedure, we should choose to be the pig. Equality of events in the decathlon is acceptable, whereas equality of utility functions does not appear to be so. To overcome this problem, we would have to directly compare the different utility functions, which have already been ruled out.

Let me recapitulate the problems associated with EU that have been established to this point. There were practical problems in assigning a cardinal scale to our preferences. When we encountered changes in utility functions, there didn't appear to be any way to perform these inter-utility comparisons. The rejection of an indirect comparison rests on our intuitions, such as in the complacency pill example.

According to the EU model, the probabilities of the alternatives have to be known to make the necessary calculations. We don't possess most of that information in any particular case before us. Nor do we possess precise numbers to attach to the values of the outcomes. Behavioral economics demonstrates this well.

Yet the consent context is one where some of the probabilities are known. Perhaps EU should be employed in this context. Of course, one still needs to know all the probabilities of the valuable alternatives and their outcomes. Since the known probabilities are usually the medical outcomes, there might be a 30 percent chance of liver failure, remission, or something else.

Appendix C

Expected Value

Utility functions play a vital role in decision-making theory. The basic nature of these functions has been described in the court text. We have also seen that these utility functions can be at odds even within a person over time. Gambling scenarios have long been the standard basis for applying these functions in conditions of uncertainty. In our context, we are choosing between medical alternatives with different preferences over some time. Expected value calculations are intriguing in that they can provide the best answer as to how to proceed. Our requirements are a bit less stringent. We are happy with good decisions, however that might get defined.

Of course, there are many ways in which decisions can be made. Coins can be tossed, tickets drawn from a hat, a democratic vote can be taken, etc.

This type of decision-making is utilitarian in character. We have left out some important calculations required when using the utilitarian approach. In essence, we have not accounted for net gains and net losses in an explicit fashion.

The net gains and losses are represented in the following choice problem. Imagine that you must decide between two business alternatives. Say you need to make a meeting by a certain time, and you can take the train or the bus. The train costs $50. The bus costs $10. If you take the train, you have a 40 percent chance of making it early, impressing your customer, which results in a payoff of $300.

On the other hand, this choice leaves you a 60 percent chance of just being late with a payoff of -$80. The customer removes an order from you due to your tardiness. The math for net gain looks like this:

Expected Value of the train results in a 0.4 chance of a payoff of $300 and a 0.6 chance of losing $80. EV is (.4*$300)- (.6*48) = $120-$28.80 = $91.20. Ah, but we have not considered the ticket cost, which is $50. That calculation is $91.20 minus the $50 train ticket. The net gain is $41.20 if the train scenario is adopted.

Alternatively, you could take the bus. You have an 80 percent chance of only being slightly late, but it reduces the payoff with the customer to $30. You have a 20 percent chance of being 20 minutes late, reducing your payoff to $15. The math for the bus looks like this:

Expected Value of the bus results in a .8 chance payoff of $30 and a .2 chance of losing $15. The EV for the bus is (.8*$30) – (.2*$15). The EV is ($24-$3) = $21. The net gain for the bus is the EV minus the cost, which is the $10 ticket. The net gain for the bus is $21 - $10 = $11. When comparing the two modes of transportation, the net gain for the train is better.

Generalized Formulation of EV

The figure below is a generalized version of the EV model. Individual X is confronted initially with alternatives A1 and A1'. As time passes, other decision points go from left to right. The probabilities at each juncture should equal 1.

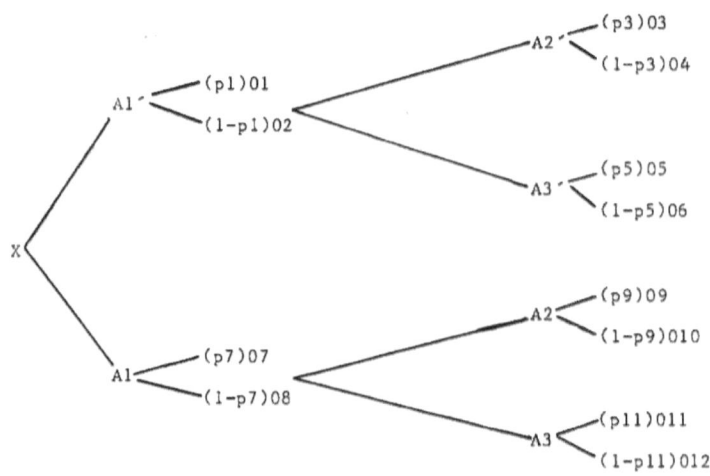

Figure 3 EU formulas in a decision tree

The expected utility for alternative Al' would be pl x (u)Ol +(l-pl) x (u)O2, where pl is the probability associated with outcome O1 and (1-p1) is the probability associated with the outcome for O2. The (u)Ol and (u)O2 are the values assigned by a utility function (u) to outcomes O1 and O2, respectively.

In this figure, the person represents the decision maker and Al, A2, Al', A2', etc. represent different alternatives. Initially, the person has to choose between alternatives Al and Al'. Suppose you must choose between these two alternatives. Suppose the person chooses A2 and so on until the person dies. This way, the person will have chosen an entire sequence of alternatives among all possible sequences. (So as not to be misleading, it should be stated that there may be more than two alternatives at any point in time and that any one alternative may be available at different times. The figure is for illustration only.)

As stated, the problem confronting the person is choosing the best alternative at time t1. Part of what this entails is choosing the best sequence. For example, suppose that Al' in and of itself were better than Al, but A2' and A3' were very poor alternatives compared to either A2 or A3. In a case such as this, it may be that alternative Al should be chosen because the sequences which follow are better than those which follow Al'. In fact, the person is trying to pick the best sequence of alternatives.

A concrete example may help to illustrate this point. When I receive my paycheck every two weeks, I could spend it all on payday (Al') or about 10 percent (Al). On payday, Al' is better than Al, which captures one thing we might mean by choosing the better alternative. But it is also rather clear that if I select Al', then the following sequences of alternatives are dismal. The sequences that follow from Al are much better and yield a more favorable outcome overall. In this sense, Al is better than Al'. It is this latter sense that is appropriate to the purpose at hand.

This presents the first major issue in clarifying the act of decision-making. If the person decides that one sequence is better than another, then the person must have a way of assigning a value to each outcome, alternative, and sequence. Technically, the person employs a utility function (U) which assigns a value to each of the outcomes and calculates an expected utility for each alternative (see Figure 3).

The type of utility function chosen plays a crucial role in determining which alternatives and sequences are best. It is also the case that different utility functions have different epistemological characteristics. Because of this, I have divided the utility functions into two types according to epistemological considerations. According to this type of division, utility functions are either objective or subjective.

Objective utility functions do not vary from one individual's set of preferences to another's. We do not have to know what an individual prefers to know the objective utility function for them.

One example of this type of function would have the medical alternatives evaluated based on physiological functioning. Suppose Al will restore full physiological function in one week but will cause intense pain. Al' will gradually restore physiological function over two months, but without pain. The utility function based on physiological function alone will yield that Al is better than Al'. The objective utility function, in general, will assign a value to a state of the individual (alternative) without regard for how that individual might value that alternative (state). Of course, the individual could value these states as the objective function does. They could coincide.

The individual generates subjective utility functions in some way. An individual's verbally expressed preferences would be one such function, while an individual's behaviorally expressed preferences could be another. Some others include happiness, pleasure, and other experiential states.

The subjective functions could yield an entirely different result in the medical example. The patient's happiness would probably be (though not necessarily) better served by choosing Al'. The key point is that the individual generates the preference scale.

The two types of functions have vastly different epistemological characteristics, as mentioned. The objective functions can be determined by parties other than the patient. Everyone has equal access, as it were. There is no need to know anything about the patient's preference system to know how values will be assigned to the alternatives.

The subjective functions, by definition, necessitate knowledge of the patient's preference system. The patient, more often than not, will have better access than anyone else to that preference system.

The question arises regarding which of these utility functions is appropriate in this context. The answer lies at the interface between the moral and epistemological aspects of the consent situation. This means I will have to take a slight diversion into the moral realm of the consent situation.

Moral considerations necessitate the consent of the patient. Patients are regarded as autonomous beings with a right to that autonomy. Patients have a right to direct and determine their fate. Consequently, the medical community cannot take it into its own hands as to which alternative should be pursued. If the medical community had made a choice, the patient's right would have been violated. Therefore, the patient has to give· consent for any medical intervention being considered.

An interesting and important feature of this social practice is that not all patients have this right to self-determination. Individuals who are excluded include the following: the insane, the senile, the comatose, young children, the severely retarded, and possibly others. It would be of great importance if these individuals lacked some characteristics necessary for being included in the practice.

The characteristic most often proposed is that of competency. Competency is perceived to be a necessary condition for autonomy. It has not been made clear, to my knowledge, as to why this is so, but there is a good justification for it. This justification provides the conceptual tie between morality and the epistemology of consent.

The right that the individual enjoys is that of the right to self-determination and self-direction, or autonomy. It is difficult to say exactly what these concepts entail, but we can draw some rough conclusions. These conclusions sufficiently clarify the connection between competency and consent to choose between objective utility and subjective functions.

Individuals who direct and determine their own lives cause and control their destinies as much as is humanly possible. They are not merely swept along in a mechanistic causal chain that is (thought to be) external to them. They influence what will happen to them and who they will be. Both activities (self-direction and self- determination) come under the broad umbrella of autonomy.

The degree to which individuals are able to direct and determine themselves is unquestionably dependent upon several variables. Among these are the following abilities: an understanding of the available alternatives; knowing the likelihood of the various outcomes; evaluating the merits of the alternatives and their consequences; and choosing the alternative with the most merit.

These abilities can be perceived as internal mental abilities. They form part of the self and, as such, remove the person's mental activity from the external succession of events. They are part of the "self" portion of self-direction and self-determination. However, that is only part of the story since certain internal happenings can make an individual just as bound to a causal juggernaut as any "external" cause. Some people cannot but follow their impulses and, as such, are not considered to be autonomous.

Another feature of the abilities cited above is that these abilities are goal-directed or teleological. As such, they bring us out of a blind mechanistic causal system. They form the "directing" part of self-direction. Since these abilities also constitute part of our rational nature, it is not surprising to make a connection between our freedom and our rationality.

This self-direction feature presumably enables us to overcome being forced to act only according to our impulses. I suspect that it is any mechanistic causal chain that is being overcome by our autonomy, whether the causes be internal or external. Whether or not this metaphysical sketch of autonomy is correct is beyond our scope.

It does provide a way of connecting the moral and epistemological elements of the social practice of obtaining consent.

Assuming that the line of argument above is correct, the abilities listed above form part of our concept of autonomy. They also form part of our concept of the competent decision-maker. The connection between the two concepts is a logical one. The concepts overlap, and it appears that one could not be autonomous without being competent at decision-making (it is unclear about the contrary proposition).

At this point, the moral aspect of the situation can be clarified to some extent. The moral issue is, who has the right to select the alternative? The act of selection can result from many different methods (as pointed out earlier). One need not be competent or autonomous to make a selection. It is the act of selection that is under dispute. (More appropriately, it is who has the right to make the selection that is under dispute.) We presume that only autonomous decision-makers should have the right to perform the act of autonomous selection.

The argument for this position is as follows: A person has the right to do A only if the person has the ability to do A. Otherwise, the person would be unable to exercise the right under any circumstances, and it does seem nonsensical to ascribe a right to someone who does not have the ability to exercise it.

What can be misleading, in this case, is that the act of selection can be part of an autonomous or non-autonomous act. A person may not have the ability to select autonomously but could still have the ability to select in a non-autonomous fashion; the non-autonomous selector would not, indeed could not, have the right to make the autonomous selection because the ability to do so would not be present, Consequently, not allowing such a person to make the selection would not violate any right, since this person did not possess the right in the first place. There may be other reasons for allowing non-autonomous people the right to select, based on some utilitarian notions.

This argument provides a rationale for excluding the senile, children, individuals with mental disabilities, and the comatose from the right to select; the right to select is perceived as part of the right to autonomy. People who aren't competent aren't autonomous and cannot, conceptually, possess the right to self-determination. Consequently, they have no right to make the selection. I want to emphasize that there may be utilitarian grounds for permitting some of these people to make their selections.

Given this rationale for ascribing the right of autonomy to patients, it follows that a subjective utility function should be employed. Only if the patient's preference system is employed can the act be taken as self-directed and self-determined.

Let us give a bit of a recap of the informed consent paradigm and its problems. We have set out two goals for the paradigms for the activity with the patient. The goals are to protect the patient's right to self-determination, otherwise called "autonomy." The second goal and secondary goals were to promote good decision-making. We will focus on how the right to self-determination can lead to the idea of making good decisions.

We saw way back at the beginning from the diner examples that having knowledge helps us to be in some control of the situation. Blindly selecting options doesn't feel like much control. The ethical point of view would say that respect for autonomy can narrowly be defined by letting patients make choices. So, when we think of the rights of individuals, in this case, patients, we are saying our obligation as health care providers is to just get out of the way. It is clear that the informed consent paradigm would include more than just initially saying what you want in terms of surgery or medical intervention. It would also include more information than that. The litany of court cases pretty well demonstrated this. Why should the information be in the paradigm to this extent?

I hypothesize that the connection is due to a more robust idea of self-determination. The simplistic view of self-determination would have the individual select just what they want. There are good reasons for thinking this way, and I believe it applies to a lot of the many decisions we make in our daily lives. We are faced with myriad decisions that are simply decided upon what I want to do now. They are not momentous decisions. I have three grocery stores in which I can shop. Two have similar pricing and are about the same distance from my house. One has better meats, and the other has better produce, and I need both. The third grocery store is further away and costs more but has better meat and produce. Where shall I go? Right now, I don't feel like going the extra distance, and now I'm more interested in the produce for no good reason. So, I go to the second grocery store. I'm not imagining much down the road in the future, saving money, calculating the difference in gas consumption and prices, and so on. I start doing that, and I'll soon be going hungry. Some things I want, and I want them now.

This certainly is a free choice on my part, and in some sense, I am determining my immediate future and the consequences of these actions that I will experience down the road. This can be distinguished from those cases of immediate and delayed gratification. We can look at children and offer them pieces of candy, chocolate preferable, and say I offer them one piece now, or they can choose to have two pieces in 20 minutes. Children recognize the difference and the amount. Experimental studies show that most children will choose the one piece now, but a subset will learn to delay and have more enjoyment later. Do we consider immediate gratifiers to be less autonomous than those who can delay gratification? While we do use the term self-control quite a bit in this regard, typically, it means that we can determine for ourselves more freely than not.

This coincides well with the diner examples. When receiving more relevant information, there is more of a feeling of being in control of the situation. This makes it arguably part of their gratification of the paradigm. The consent has to be informed to be an exercise in self-determination. In ethical jargon and frameworks, we are concerned with our duties and obligations toward patients. It is easier to frame the issue as one of respecting autonomy. We don't really talk about respecting self-determination.

Portraying the issue as one of self-determination more easily leads to the informed consent paradigm, including the assistance toward that self-determination. It makes more sense as to why the informed consent paradigm failed.

Working backward from these two requirements, certain things will follow. The relevance of the information to be disseminated can only be guessed if the patient is not involved in what's important. The court cases and the diner examples certainly bear this out. It is not the whole story if we believe in self-determination; it's part and parcel required of a working paradigm. What else does self-determination require in this situation?

We saw that the patient's values and preferences are critical in the process. How does that relate to self-determination? Here is where things could go deep into philosophical weeds. I do not intend to go that deep. However, this is how I think it would go. We are assuming in the paradigm the nature of who I am it's related to how I prefer things. The choices I make that are important are based on my actual preferences. Alternatively, it might be based on what I think is my actual preference. Finally, it could be based on what I think should be my preferences. In this decision-making context, my sense of self is related to my preference structure. The Self in self-determination is mine. It is my preference structure that is the important one. It isn't the physician's preference structure that plays a role.

This establishes the connection between the values required and the paradigm of informed consent. The values are needed to support self-determination. There really is a two-way street here. On the one hand, the patient's values will instruct the health care professional about the relevant information types. This is in service to supporting self-determination. Clarifying the patient's preference structure will also serve self-determination by clarifying the nature of those values. Informed consent played no interest in patient values. It was as if they were off-limits. The major focus of the informed consent paradigm was the information provided by the health care professional. It failed.

What about shared decision-making? It has answers to some of the challenges of informed consent. It shines a light on the patient and the information the patient has to share. That information can guide the health care professional on what medical data is important and relevant. Shining the light on the patient has added to the shared decision-making paradigm. It has added weight to the idea of self-determination. The self has a preference structure and requires some assistance. This makes sense of the increased research on values clarification.

The decision-making procedure is another major component of the paradigm to be discussed. Is this part of the paradigm or not? If we are to take self-determination seriously as part of the paradigm, then this follows suit. The point of the exercise from a patient's point of view is not only to get good information from the health care provider. That is just a means to my end. My end is to achieve the best goals for myself as possible. Those goals are defined by me and not by society. I require more than just the medical information and the information that is my preference. I need a way of combining those two to make a reasonably good decision that will give me good results as defined by my value system. That this is part of the paradigm, I believe, is displayed by Judge Cardozo's ruling that required a sound mind (a very low bar) to the various arguments about paternalistic intervention, such as in the case of Dax Cowart. It plays such a prominent role in arguments about who should make the decision that it should be in the paradigm.

We briefly investigated three approaches to decision-making. They are all meant to get us where we want to be. That landing spot satisfies one's preferences. There are requirements placed on each one. Each one needs to address decision-making under uncertainty. All of them do that. They need to be practical. Expected value approaches are severely limited in this regard. Their reliance on quantifiable values (cardinal) requires us to quantify our own value system so that precision is lost. There are other theoretical limitations, such as when to stop calculating. Well, this is not the place for it. One could argue that introducing stopping rules is tantamount to sneaking in a fast and frugal methodology.

A modified Bentham approach has a lot going for it. The original model is not practical because it offers no details or instructions about performing what is called "hedonistic calculus." It does sketch out in a broad outline what I think is accurate. It does categorize what is important to be considered when making a decision. Likelihoods are important to consider when they are quite distinct. When they are not very different, they can be ignored. It would be a difference that we cannot account for when the likelihoods are close. You can think about the stadium examples. Imagine that I tell you out of the 100,000 people in this stadium, forty-nine would suffer a headache, and 50 would suffer a sore throat. In my mind, they're the same.

This could be said with the intensity of outcomes as well. On a pain scale of zero to ten, I cannot distinguish a four from a five. I can distinguish a two from an eight. I used to think of one in these circumstances, which is, of course, a way of making comparisons.

The practicality of the Bentham approach is significant. The fairness of the consequences plays a role that is not well accounted for in the expected value approach. The farther away it is, the more it gets discounted under the Bentham view. This makes it possible to put an end to the branches of the decision tree.

I have wondered whether this transforms Bentham's utilitarianism into a Fast and Frugal process. What is intriguing about fast and frugal (bounded rationality) is that it aims to be practical but also scientifically worthy. There may be algorithms to suggest what stopping rules would apply in these circumstances. Some literature indicates that Fast and Frugal is not particularly applicable to this environment, but I am not sure it can't be. There may be a good algorithm for clarification of values. Making a list and ordering items by location on the list could be a clue as to the order of importance for a person. It would need to be tested, of course.

The shared decision-making paradigm overcomes the issue that led to the failure of the informed consent paradigm. This does not mean it is developed enough to satisfy the two goals that any of these approaches are meant to accomplish. What issues remain to be addressed? Let's have at it.

Looking at the large landscape from a distance, this decision-making apparatus and processes need to be fleshed out. The concern is that if we make the decision-making process too difficult to perform, we will unnecessarily weed out a majority of the adult population from making their own decisions. Frankly, it's an argument for abandoning the expected value model. There are other arguments that we have made to abandon it as well, including the issue of quantifying values. So let us frame the challenge appropriately. Rational decision-making that supports self-determination requires more than the ability to point to an alternative on a list. It requires less than an advanced degree in statistical analysis. We know it lies somewhere between these two extremes to fit the required paradigm. It needs to be practical, so the way lends itself to a Fast and Frugal approach and a modified Benthamite model. Is there something more we can say?

We know that our thinking about choices is fraught with difficulty in the real world. Everyone, including statisticians and behavioral economists, is subject to the same types of errors. Much of the above approaches to statistical information are meant to either remove the issue or at least minimize it. The fact that we view losses as being more important than gains makes us more protective of where we are than willing to take chances of where we could be. As an example, I recently injured my right hand, which is not functional at the moment.

Consequently, I have learned to use my left hand quite a bit. I bemoan the loss of this temporary functionality more than I value the gain, which may be more long-term, in my left-hand dexterity and strength. There have been enough behavioral economic experiments to show that a loss of money versus a gain of an equivalent amount is more important. Our valuations follow the prospect theory curve of Kahneman and Tversky. This becomes critically important in how to package information to patients. I can express your likelihood of surviving two years or your mortality in the same length. If you are like most people, the information feels different if it is framed as a survival rate versus the mortality rate. It is just the way it is. I suspect that hearing the information connects with a whole series of other coherent thoughts. If you talk about mortality, I am conjuring up the end of my life, fear, and anxiety. If you're talking about survival, I'll think about being alive. I definitely have two different feelings about those two different states. Sometimes prospect theory is also called loss aversion. The idea is that we'd be willing to do more to avert the loss. One could hypothesize that patients would be more willing to be treated than if the positive survival rate were transmitted.

This problem of describing the container of information has left me somewhat perplexed. In some cases, we could describe the situation both positively and negatively. Either portrayal is valid. Since our valuing is based on our thinking one perspective, it is subject to this inconsistency.

Prospect theory involves reference points. We can alter our judgments based on reference points rather than absolute measures. It requires the patient to imagine or recall an experience similar to what they may encounter. This relates to the idea of the relative starting point for an individual. It has similar markings to marginal utilities. It follows the pattern we would use to compare the intensities of events to heights. We have a starting point to which we refer. In gambles, the reference point can be the bet or how rich I happen to be. Let's take someone else who is actually rich. They may be willing to lose a $1000 bet without blinking an eye. The loss of version only hits them once we're in the hundreds of thousands of potential losses. Compared to my reference point, I don't want to lose anything.

Typically, more than one or two alternatives are available for important decisions. At the very least, they should all be described in either a positive or negative manner. Describing the alternatives consistently as either positive or negative is important. Patients will be able to skew the alternatives the same way. No alternative gains an advantage.

A shared decision-making paradigm would need to address numerous specific pitfalls in our decision-making apparatus. This is evident once we agree that the paradigm's goal is to support the patient's self-determination. Health care professionals would be obligated to find ways to support self-determination. Part of this is the values clarification that already exists in the paradigm demonstrated by the research that is published. Health literacy is another avenue that is being explored.

Like Gigerenzer and others, what has already begun is the exploration of fast and frugal methods for decision-making itself. Their take on this endeavor is to look for the cues to bring about successful results. It is certainly not clear at this juncture of paradigm development how successful this will be or whether it can be subsumed under a more modified Bentham-like approach. We can say that whatever method is used, it must be more practical than 100 branches off a decision tree. It also can only involve a small amount of time on behalf of the health care team to move on. As patients, we won't perform that way anyway, and we certainly have more of a shared sense of values than the literature would suggest for many of our health care decisions.

We can sketch out this modified Bentham version to look something like this. Patients and physicians have a general discussion about the choices that are available to them. Patients can inform their physicians through some sort of values clarification in broad terms; these are the categories of interest for them. That will spark the physicians to relay the appropriate types of information relevant to what the patient has expressed. This certainly will only be for some encounters. The decisions involve making differential diagnoses and what would be involved. I do not need to map out my personal campaign to get any of this done. I came here for relief from a certain condition. The physician has told me what alternatives would provide me some relief and the most frequent or serious side effects. None of these would be particularly eye-opening. Sometimes we lose sight of the interaction's purpose when discussing the relationship's philosophical bases and ethical components. Manson and O'Neill have written quite persuasively on this topic. There are, however, certain situations that warrant the extra time to be devoted to the discussion. It is really a Fast and Frugal approach to the whole area of informing in medical encounters.

The components that I would want to gather for this Bentham approach are the likelihood of positive and negative events occurring within a limited time frame and a limited number of alternatives. The propinquity (I love that word) of the consequences needs to be near the middle term. Going 20 years down the road isn't helpful unless it's incredibly serious. We could explain to professional athletes at the beginning of their careers that they will suffer broken bones and joint problems later in life. Some of them will get arthritis and have difficulty walking. In American football, there need to be warnings about concussions and their potentially devastating effects, which may occur 40 years later. On the other hand, we wouldn't want to go through the later effects of a bone bruise. It is unlikely to have any serious implications 20 years from now.

The likelihoods really apply when there are significant differences between them. Eight percent versus 10 percent is simply not calculable in our Think1 state. We will default to thinking they're the same. In essence, the precision problem for EV is handled by the fact that we seriously round on the probability side just as we do on the value side.

The calculations we make need to be quite simple to be successful. A strategy that may be employed in shared decision-making in the future is to limit the alternatives being presented after discussion and a values clarification. Too much information clouds what's important. The values clarification can also instruct on the order of presentation of alternatives. Important items are presented first and perhaps repeated at the end. This should reinforce the patient's value preferences, not the health care professionals.

We have thus modified Bentham's approach by giving ourselves a stopping rule for the calculation based on propinquity. We will still be combining the likelihood of an outcome with its value. I imagine that this really means that the likelihood creates a certain level of intensity to be combined with the intensity of the value somebody has. In essence, it'll be a rank ordering rather than a cardinal ordering. It is really all that's needed for these decisions. You choose the alternative that came to mind first.

Works Cited

Ariely, Dan. Predictably Irrational: The Hidden Forces That Shape Our Decisions. HarperCollins, 2009.

Arrow, Kenneth J. *Social Choice and Individual Values: Third Edition*. 3rd ed., Yale University Press, 2012.

Aune, Bruce. "Can." *Encyclopedia of Philosophy*, MacMillan Publishing Co, 1967, pp. 18–20.

Baker, M. T. "Readability of Informed Consent Forms for Research in a Veterans Administration Medical Center." *JAMA: The Journal of the American Medical Association*, vol. 250, no. 19, 1983, pp. 2646–2648, https://doi.org10.1001/jama.250.19.2646.

Barrow, John. "Decathlon: The Art of Scoring Points." *Sport.maths.org*, 2013, https://sport.maths.or/content/decathalon-art-scoring-points-0.

Bateson, Melissa, et al. "Cues of Being Watched Enhance Cooperation in a Real-World Setting." *Biology Letters*, vol. 2, no. 3, 2006, pp. 412–414, https://doi.org10.1098/rsbl.2006.0509.

Beck, Lewis W., and Immanuel Kant. *Foundations of the Metaphysics of Morals and What Is Enlightenment? Kant*. Prentice Hall, 1959.

Benson, Buster. "Cognitive Bias Cheat Sheet." *Medium: Better Humans*, ep 1 2016, https://medium.com/better-humans/cognitive-bias-cheat-sheet-55a472476b18.

Bentham, Jeremy. *An Introduction to the Principles of Morals and Legislation.* Dover Publications, 2012.

Biser, Erwin. "Physics and Microphysics. Louis DeBroglie. Translated by Martin Davidson with a Foreword by Albert Einstein. New York: Pantheon Books, 1955. Pp. 286. $4.50." *Philosophy of Science*, vol. 24, no. 3, 1957, pp. 281–282, https://doi.org10.1086/287544.

Blumenthal-Barby, Jennifer S. *Good Ethics and Bad Choices: The Relevance of Behavioral Economics for Medical Ethics.* MIT Press, 2021.

Brand, Myles. *The Nature of Human Action.* Scott Foresman, 1970.

Bricker, Phillip. "Prudence." *Journal of Philosophy,* vol. 77, no. 7, 1980, pp. 381-401.

"Canterbury v Spence." *464 F.2d,* vol. D. C. Cir, 1972, p. 772.

Choudhary, Rahul, and David Blair. "All Possible Paths: Bringing Quantum Electrodynamics to Classrooms." *European Journal of Physics*, vol. 42, no. 3, 2021, p. 035408, https://doi.org10.1088/1361-6404/abef5b.

"Cobbs v. Grant." *8 Cal 3d.*, vol. 104 Cal. Rptr. 505,502 P 2d, 1972, p. 229.

Conant, James Bryant. *Harvard Case Histories in Experimental Science Volume I.* Nabu Press, 2013.

Dax Cowart Compilation. Vmeo, 2016, https://vimeo.com/164747014.

deBroglie, Louis. *Interpretation of Quantum Mechanics by the Double Solution Theory.* 1987, https://fondationlouisdebroglie.org.

Declaration of Helsinki 2013. Canary Publications, 2020

Deniz, Serkan, et al. "The Mediating Role of Shared Decision-Making in the Effect of the Patient-Physician Relationship on Compliance with Treatment." *Journal of Patient Experience*, vol. 8, 2021, p. 23743735211018064, https://doi.org10.1177/23743735211018066.

Edwards, Adrian, and Glyn Elwyn, editors. *Shared Decision-Making in Health Care: Achieving Evidence-Based Patient Choice*. Oxford University Press, 2009.

Elster, Jon, editor. *Ulysses and the Sirens: Studies in Rationality and Irrationality*. Cambridge University Press, 1984.

Elster, Jon. *Sour Grapes: Studies in the Subversion of Rationality*. Cambridge University Press, 1985.

Elwyn, Glyn. "Shared Decision Making: What Is the Work?" *Patient Education and Counseling*, vol. 104, no. 7, 2021, pp. 1591–1595, https://doi.org10.1016/j.pec.2020.11.032.

Feynman, Richard P., and A. R. Hibbs. *Quantum Mechanics and Path Integrals*. McGraw-Hill, 1965.

Gigerenzer, Gerd. *Gut Feelings: Short Cuts to Better Decision Making*. Penguin Books, 2008.

—. Risk Savvy: How to Make Good Decisions. Allen Lane, 2005.

Gigerenzer, Gerd, and Wolfgang Gaissmaier. "Heuristic Decision Making." *Annual Review of Psychology*, vol. 62, no. 1, 2011, pp. 451–482, https://doi.org10.1146/annurev-psych-120709-145346.

Gladwell, Malcolm. *Blink: The Power of Thinking without Thinking*. Penguin Books, 2006.

Glaser, Johanna, et al. "Interventions to Improve Patient Comprehension in Informed Consent for Medical and Surgical Procedures: An Updated Systematic Review." *Medical Decision Making: An International Journal of the Society for Medical Decision Making*, vol. 40, no. 2, 2020, pp. 119–143, https://doi.org10.1177/0272989X19896348.

Greenberg, R. N. "Overview of Patient Compliance with Medication Dosing: A Literature Review." *Clinical Therapeutics*, vol. 6, no. 5, 1984, pp. 592–599.

Greenfield, S., et al. "Expanding Patient Involvement in Care. Effects on Patient Outcomes." *Annals of Internal Medicine*, vol. 102, no. 4, 1985, pp. 520–528, https://doi.org10.7326/0003-4819-102-4-520.

Hughes et al, Tasha. "Association of Shared Decision-Making on Patient-Reported Health Outcomes and Healthcare Utilization." *American Journal of Surgery*, vol. 216, no. 1, 2018, pp. 7–12, https://doi.org10.1016/j.amjsurg.2018.01.011.

Hume, David. *An Enquiry Concerning Human Understanding*. Dover Publications, 2004.

James, William. *The Principles of Psychology Volumes 1 and 2*. 2011th ed., Digireads.com, 2011.

"Judith Jarvis Thomson (1971), 'A Defense of Abortion', Philosophy and Public Affairs, 1, Pp. 47-66." *Abortion*, Routledge, 2017, pp. 27–46.

Kahneman, Daniel. *Thinking, Fast and Slow*. eBook Penguin Books, 2012.

Kaplan, Sherrie H., et al. "Assessing the Effects of Physician-Patient Interactions on the Outcomes of Chronic Disease." *Medical Care*, vol. 27, no. Supplement, 1989, pp. S110–S127, https://doi.org10.1097/00005650-198903001-00010.

Katz, Jay, and M.D. *The Silent World of Doctor and Patient*. Free Press, 1986.

King, Jaime Staples, and Benjamin W. Moulton. "Rethinking Informed Consent: The Case for Shared Medical Decision-Making." *American Journal of Law & Medicine*, vol. 32, no. 4, 2006, pp. 429–501, https://doi.org10.1177/009885880603200401.

Kaufman, A. S. "Ability." *The Nature of Human Action*, edited by Myles Brand, Scott Foresman and Co, 1970, p. 199.

King, Jaime Staples, and Benjamin W. Moulton. "Rethinking Informed Consent: The Case for Shared Medical Decision-Making." *American Journal of Law & Medicine*, vol. 32, no. 4, 2006, pp. 429–501, https://doi.org10.1177/009885880603200401.

Kuhn, Thomas S. *The Structure of Scientific Revolutions*. 2nd ed., Books on Demand, 1970.

Locke, Don. "The 'Can' of Being Able." *Philosophia*, vol. 6, no. 1, 1974, pp. 1–2.

Mackay, A. Arrow's Theorem, the Paradox of Social Choice: A Case Study in the Philosophy of Economics. Yale University Press, 1980.

Manson, Neil C., and Onora O'Neill. *Rethinking Informed Consent in Bioethics*. Cambridge University Press, 2007.

McCullough, Laurence B., et al. "Perils of Miscommunication: The Beginnings of Informed Consent." *Donald School Journal of Ultrasound in Obstetrics & Gynecology*, vol. 10, no. 2, 2016, pp. 125–130, https://doi.org10.5005/jp-journals-10009-1454.

Mill, J.S. *A System of Logic, Ratiocinative and Inductive*. eBook Harper & Brothers. 1882

Miller, Robert. *Unpublished Monographs by Robert D. Miller Slater v. Baker and Stapleton Monograph #2*. https://minds.wisconsin.edu/handle/1793/80595.

Morris, Charles. *The San Francisco Calamity*. AUK Academic and Technical, 2012.

"Natanson v Kline." *186 Kan*, vol. 350 P.2d 1093, 1960, p. 393. ebook

Open Science Collaboration. "Estimating the Reproducibility of Psychological Science." *Science (New York, N.Y.)*, vol. 349, no. 6251, 2015, pp. aac4716–aac4716, https://doi.org10.1126/science.aac4716.

Parfit, Derek. *Reasons and Persons*. Oxford University Press, 1986.

Pascal, Blaise. *Pensées*. Translated by W. F. Trotter, Dover Publications, 2003.

Pietrzykowski, Tomasz, and Katarzyna Smilowska. "The Reality of Informed Consent: Empirical Studies on Patient Comprehension-Systematic Review." *Trials*, vol. 22, no. 1, 2021, p. 57, https://doi.org10.1186/s13063-020-04969-w.

President's Commission for the Study of Ethical Problems in Medicine and Biomedical and Behavioral. *Making Health Care Decisions*. Government Printing Office, 1982.

Richards, J., and P. McDonald. "Doctor-Patient Communication in Surgery." *Journal of the Royal Society of Medicine*, vol. 78, no. 11, 1985, pp. 922–924, https://doi.org10.1177/014107688507801109.

"Salgo v Leland Stanford Jr. University Board of Trustees." *154 Cal App. 2d*, vol. 317 P.2d 170, 1957, p. 560.

"Schloendorff v Society of N.Y. Hospital (Transcript of Testimony. Number Refer to Paragraph Number)." *105 N.E. 92*, vol. 93 N.Y., 1914, p. 93.

Sen, Amartya, and Bernard Williams, editors. *Utilitarianism and Beyond*. Cambridge University Press, 2011.

Simon, Herbert A. "A Behavioral Model of Rational Choice." *The Quarterly Journal of Economics*, vol. 69, no. 1, 1955, p. 99, https://doi.org10.2307/1884852.

"Slater v Baker and Stapleton." *Eng Rep 95*, vol. E.R., 1767, p. 860.

Thornton, J. G. et al. "Decision Analysis in Medicine." *BMJ (Clinical Research Ed.*, vol. 304, no. 6834, 1992, pp. 1099–1103.

Tversky, Amos, and Daniel Kahneman. "Rational Choice and the Framing of Decisions." *The Journal of Business*, vol. 59, no. S4, 1986, p. S251, https://doi.org10.1086/296365.

Wegwarth, Odette, et al. "Deceiving Numbers: Survival Rates and Their Impact on Doctors' Risk Communication: Survival Rates and Their Impact on Doctors' Risk Communication." *Medical Decision Making: An International Journal of the Society for Medical Decision Making*, vol. 31, no. 3, 2011, pp. 386–394, https://doi.org10.1177/0272989X10391469.

Whitman, Walt. *Leaves of Grass: Original Edition*. Independently Published, 2021.

Witteman, Holly O., et al. "Clarifying Values: An Updated and Expanded Systematic Review and Meta-Analysis." *Medical Decision Making: An International Journal of the Society for Medical Decision Making*, vol. 41, no. 7, 2021, pp. 801–820, https://doi.org10.1177/0272989X211037946.

Suggested Readings

Beauchamp, and Childress. *Principles of Biomedical Ethics*. 8th ed., Oxford University Press, 2019.

Bomhof-Roordink, Hanna, et al. "Key Components of Shared Decision Making Models: A Systematic Review." *BMJ Open*, vol. 9, no. 12, 2019, p. e031763, https://doi.org10.1136/bmjopen-2019-031763.

Childress, James F., and Marcia Day Childress. "What Does the Evolution from Informed Consent to Shared Decision Making Teach Us about Authority in Health Care?" *AMA Journal of Ethics*, vol. 22, no. 5, 2020, pp. E423-429, https://doi.org10.1001/amajethics.2020.423.

Elwyn, Glyn, Dominick L. Frosch, et al. "Implementing Shared Decision-Making: Consider All the Consequences." *Implementation Science: IS*, vol. 11, no. 1, 2016, p. 114, https://doi.org10.1186/s13012-016-0480-9.

Elwyn, Glyn, Dominick Frosch, et al. "Shared Decision Making: A Model for Clinical Practice." *Journal of General Internal Medicine*, vol. 27, no. 10, 2012, pp. 1361–1367, https://doi.org10.1007/s11606-012-2077-6.

Frosch, D. L., and R. M. Kaplan. "Shared Decision Making in Clinical Medicine: Past Research and Future Directions." *American Journal of Preventive Medicine*, vol. 17, no. 4, 1999, pp. 285–294, https://doi.org10.1016/s0749-3797(99)00097-5.

Gert, Bernard, et al. *Bioethics: A Systematic Approach*. 2nd ed., Oxford University Press, 2006.

Gigerenzer, Gerd, and J. A. Muir Gray, editors. *Better Doctors, Better Patients, Better Decisions: Envisioning Health Care 2020*. The MIT Press, 2011.

Kant, Immanuel. *Critique of Practical Reason*. Translated by Thomas K. Abbott, Dover Publications, 2004.

Levere, Trevor H. Transforming Matter: A History of Chemistry from Alchemy to the Buckyball. Johns Hopkins University Press, 2003.

McCullough, Laurence B., et al. "Perils of Miscommunication: The Beginnings of Informed Consent." *Donald School Journal of Ultrasound in Obstetrics & Gynecology*, vol. 10, no. 2, 2016, pp. 125–130, https://doi.org10.5005/jp-journals-10009-1454.

Mill, John Stuart. *Utilitarianism*. Phoenix, 1993.

Raab, Markus, and Gerd Gigerenzer. "The Power of Simplicity: A Fast-and-Frugal Heuristics Approach to Performance Science." *Frontiers in Psychology*, vol. 6, 2015, p. 1672, https://doi.org10.3389/fpsyg.2015.01672.

Saheb Kashaf, Michael, et al. "Shared Decision-Making and Outcomes in Type 2 Diabetes: A Systematic Review and Meta-Analysis." *Patient Education and Counseling*, vol. 100, no. 12, 2017, pp. 2159–2171, https://doi.org10.1016/j.pec.2017.06.030.

Shay, L. Aubree, and Jennifer Elston Lafata. "Where Is the Evidence? A Systematic Review of Shared Decision Making and Patient Outcomes." *Medical Decision Making: An International Journal of the Society for Medical Decision Making*, vol. 35, no. 1, 2015, pp. 114–131, https://doi.org10.1177/0272989X14551638.

Wear, Stephen. Informed Consent: Patient Autonomy and Physician Beneficence within Clinical Medicine. Springer, 2010.

White, Becky Cox. *Competence to Consent*. Edited by Becky Cox White, Georgetown University Press, 1994.

Index

About the Author

Steven Kahn is a consultant in the life sciences. He received his PhD in philosophy and has a career that has spanned teaching university courses in bioethics, bedside nursing, chair of an ethics consultation committee, and providing design, implementation and oversight for safety studies in biopharmaceutical research.

He can be reached at info@TheParadigmLens.com. You can visit more of Dr. Kahn's work on the website theparadigmlens.com.

www.ingramcontent.com/pod-product-compliance
Lightning Source LLC
Chambersburg PA
CBHW020243130626
46549CB00005B/2038